A Study on Handgrip Strength in Patients With Type 2 Diabetes Mellitus

By

Ravneet Sandhu

Copyright©2022

Book Name: *A Study on Handgrip Strength in Patients With Type 2 Diabetes Mellitus*

ABSTRACT

The purpose of the present study was to observe the effect of type-2 diabetes mellitus on handgrip strength in males and females of Amritsar, Punjab and to search any relationship of handgrip strength with 22 anthropometric variables in them.

Study group consisted of 576 confirmed cases of type-2 diabetes mellitus (251 males, 325 females) with a mean duration of diabetes of more than 5 years, and 529 controls (241 males, 288 females) without any history of glucose intolerance from Amritsar, Punjab. The subjects ranged from age group of 30-65 years. A total of 1072 (97.05%) samples studied were right hand dominant. The subjects were taken from the rural and urban belt of Amritsar. The subjects' age was estimated from their birth date. The data was collected from Civil Hospital Amritsar, Civil Hospital Ajnala, Dr. Rohit Kapoor's Clinic, Rani Ka Bagh and Camp at Attari. Before the commencement of the study, the subjects were made aware about the study and a written consent was obtained. Approval for the study was provided by the institutional ethical committee.

Other than the evaluation of dominant and non-dominant handgrip strength, as many as 22 anthropometric variables namely height vertex, body weight, body mass index, upper arm, waist and hip circumference, biceps and triceps skinfold, upper arm, forearm and total arm length, hand length, breadth and span, arm muscle girth, arm muscle area, arm area, arm fat area, arm fat index, waist to hip ratio, % body fat and % lean body mass were measured. Standard techniques given by Lohmann *et al.* (1988) were followed to take all the anthropometric measurements on each subject.

In the present study, statistically significant differences ($p<0.03$-0.001) were observed in dominant and non-dominant handgrip strength, age, upper arm, waist and hip circumference, biceps and triceps skinfold, arm muscle girth, arm muscle area, arm area and arm fat area between the patients with type-2 diabetes mellitus and controls.

In the present study, significant reduction ($p\leq0.001$) in dominant and non-dominant handgrip strength was reported in diabetic males in comparison to control males. Diabetic males had significantly greater ($p\leq0.03$-0.001) mean values in age, body weight, body mass index, upper arm and hip circumference, biceps and triceps skinfold, arm area, arm fat area, arm fat index, waist to hip ratio and % body fat, and significantly lower ($p\leq0.001$) mean value of % lean body mass than their control counterparts.

Significantly lower (p<0.001) mean values of handgrip strength of both the dominant and non-dominant hand in diabetic females were noted in comparison to control females. But diabetic females had significantly greater (p≤0.01-0.001) mean values in waist circumference, triceps skinfold, arm muscle girth and arm muscle area than the control females.

In combined male and female diabetic patients, positively significant correlations (p<0.028-0.001) of dominant handgrip strength were highlighted with all the anthropometric variables studied, except age, body mass index, biceps and triceps skinfold, arm muscle girth, arm muscle area and % body fat, while negatively significant correlations (p≤0.04-0.0001) were found with age, biceps skinfold, arm muscle girth, arm muscle area and % body fat.

The correlation coefficients of non-dominant handgrip strength with selected anthropometric variables in male and female type-2 diabetic patients reported positively significant correlations (p≤0.01-0.001) with all the variables studied, except age, body mass index, biceps and triceps skinfold, arm muscle girth and % body fat, while negatively significant correlations (p≤0.046-0.001) were found with age, biceps and triceps skinfold, arm muscle girth, arm muscle area and % body fat.

Linear regression for dominant handgrip strength in combined male and female diabetic patients presented significant correlations (p<0.03-0.001) with all the anthropometric variables studied, except body mass index and triceps skinfold. For non-dominant handgrip strength in diabetic subjects, linear regression observed significant correlations (p<0.013-0.001) with all the variables studied, except body mass index and hip circumference.

The multiple regression of dominant handgrip strength with selected anthropometric variables in patients with type-2 diabetes mellitus reported significant correlations (p<0.018-0.001) with non-dominant handgrip strength, age, biceps skinfold, hand length and % lean body mass. Statistically significant correlations (p<0.001) of non-dominant handgrip strength were observed with dominant handgrip strength, total arm length and % body fat in them.

Thus, from the findings of the present study, it could be concluded that the handgrip strength was significantly affected in patients with type-2 diabetes mellitus.

TABLE OF CONTENTS

LIST OF TABLES

LIST OF FIGURES

LIST OF ABBREVIATIONS

Dhgs	:	Dominant handgrip strength
Ndhgs	:	Non-dominant handgrip strength
Hv	:	Height vertex
Bw	:	Body weight
BMI	:	Body mass index
Uac	:	Upper arm circumference
Wc	:	Waist circumference
Hc	:	Hip circumference
Bsf	:	Biceps skinfold
Tsf	:	Triceps skinfold
Ual	:	Upper arm length
Fal	:	Forearm length
Tal	:	Total arm length
Hl	:	Hand length
Hb	:	Hand breadth
Hs	:	Hand span
Amg	:	Arm muscle girth
Ama	:	Arm muscle area
Aa	:	Arm area
Afa	:	Arm fat area
Afi	:	Arm fat index
W-hr	:	Waist to hip ratio
% Bf	:	% Body fat
% Lbm	:	% Lean body mass.

INTRODUCTION

1.1 Definition

Diabetes mellitus is defined as a metabolic syndrome occurring either due to defects in insulin secretion, insulin action or both (Kumar and Clark, 2002; Beverly and Eschwege, 2003; Lindberg *et al.*, 2004). It is a heterogeneous group of disorder which results in chronic hyperglycaemia and derangements of all metabolic pathways of catabolism and anabolism of carbohydrates, lipids, proteins, minerals and water due to insulin deficiency (Shillitoe, 1988). Long standing derangements often lead to permanent or irreversible damage to body cells leading to severe diabetic complications like retinopathy (Bearse *et al.*, 2004; Hove *et al.*, 2004), neuropathy (Seki *et al.*, 2004; Moran *et al.*, 2004), nephropathy (Huang et al., 2002; Shukla *et al.*, 2003) and cardiovascular complications (Svensson *et al*, 2004; Saely, 2004).

1.2 Epidemiology

According to International Diabetes Federation (2013), type-2 diabetes mellitus affects 382 million people worldwide and expected to rise to 592 million by 2035 (Guariguata *et al.*, 2014). Diabetes Atlas estimates the number of persons with diabetes in India to rise from 40 million in 2007 to 70 million in 2025 earning the dubious distinction of "diabetes capital of the world". The highest number of diabetic patients by 2025 will be in India, China, and United States (King *et al.*, 1998; Ramachandran *et al.*, 2007). World Health Organization (1994) stated that rapid cultural and social dynamics, ageing populations, increasing urbanization, dietary changes, reduced physical activity and other unhealthy lifestyle and behavioural patterns have increased the incidence of diabetes mellitus, particularly in developing countries.

1.3 History of Diabetes Mellitus

"Madhumeha" (rain of honey) was the name given by Charak and Sushruta (600-400 B.C.) to this disease after observing the sweetness of the urine. The term Diabetes was given by Aretaeus of Cappedocia (81-138 AD) which is a Greek word meaning "to run through a siphon" due to presence of polyuria. In 1674, Thomas

Willis stated it as "pissing evil" and suggested that blood glucose levels are elevated before being excreted in urine. Thomas Cawley, in 1988, indicated the involvement of kidneys as the primary causative site of the disorder. Von Mering and Minkowski showed pancreatic extirpation (total panchreatectomy) led to the development of diabetes in dogs and diabetes related pathological changes in the islets of Langerhans of the pancreas (Warren *et al.*, 1966). Banting and Best in 1921, extracted and purified a hypoglycaemic substance "Insulin" from the pancreas of the dogs for which they were awarded the Nobel Prize (Brownlee, 1990). Chemical structure of insulin was elucidated by Sanger in 1960 and further, Radioimmunoassay (RIA) was discovered by Yalow and Berson (1960) to detect even the small amounts of insulin. Hog, bovine or porcine insulin was produced on large scale for the treatment of diabetes mellitus along with oral hypoglycaemic agents. But in the recent years with the introduction of recombinant DNA technology, large quantities of human insulin is prepared and purified using human proinsulin gene being introduced into bacterial plasmid. Nowadays, human insulin is used to treat diabetic patients.

1.4 Classification of Diabetes Mellitus

From various existing classification systems, the most widely accepted classification is given by World Health Organization (WHO) in 1980 which was initially given by Irvine (1977) and accepted by the National Diabetes Data Group (1979) and later reviewed by WHO in 1985.

1.4.1 Type-1 or Insulin dependent diabetes mellitus

Insulin dependent diabetes mellitus or juvenile onset diabetes accounts for 5-10% cases of diabetes. It occurs due to cellular mediated auto immune destruction of the β-cells of the pancreas resulting in insulin deficiency. It is clinically characterized by abrupt onset of symptoms (Gorsuch *et al.*, 1982) insulinopenia and requirement of insulin therapy for survival and tendency to develop ketoacidosis. Most of the patients demonstrate enhanced β-cell function and increase in β-cell mass immediately after the start of the insulin therapy. This period of temporary recovery may last for few months, but mostly residual β-cell function again deteriorates after 6-9 months of diagnosis of diabetes. The problems related to eyes, kidneys and nervous system present after few years of the onset of the disease. In most cases, absolute requirement of insulin therapy is required for survival. Life span of patients with insulin dependent diabetes mellitus is shortened. The patients may also develop autoimmune disorders like Grave's disease, Hashimoto's thyroiditis, Addison's disease, vitiligo, autoimmune hepatitis, myasthenia gravis and pernicious anemia.

Table 1.1: Classification of the types of diabetes mellitus (National Diabetes Data Group, 1979; World Health Organization, 1980, 1985)

Type	Characteristics
A) Type-1 or Insulin-Dependent Diabetes Mellitus (IDDM)	• Autoimmune, Idiopathic Juvenile onset, but can occur at any age β cell destruction resulting in low or absent endogenous insulin secretory capacity. • Dependent on insulin to prevent ketosis.
B) Type-2 or Non-Insulin Dependent Diabetes Mellitus (NIDDM)	• Levels of insulin may be normal, raised or deficient, characterized by hyperinsulinemia and insulin resistance; with progression of disease insulinopenia may develop. • Most of the cases do not require insulin. • Adult onset, occurs mostly after age of 40 years.
C) Gestational Diabetes Mellitus (GDM)	• Pregnancy onset glucose intolerance. • Linked with older age, obesity, family history of diabetes. • Presents higher risk for the women for development of NIDDM. • Related with higher risk of macrosomia. • Occurs in about 4% of all pregnancies.
D) Other specific types, related to:	
i) Pancreatic disease	• Due to extensive damage to pancreas by processes like pancreatitis, pancreatic reaction or cystic fibrosis.
ii) Hormonal disease	• Endocrinopathies resulting in insulin counterregulatory hormone excess (e.g., Cushing's syndrome, acromegaly).
iii) Drug or chemical exposure	• Specific drugs like glucocorticoids, pentamidine, niacin and α-interferon may lead to DM.
iv) Genetic defects	• Insulin receptor mutations or post-receptor defects. • Monogenetic defects in β-cell function.

1.4.2   Type-2 or Non- Insulin dependent diabetes mellitus

Non-insulin dependent diabetes mellitus or adult onset diabetes accounts for 90-95% of total cases of diabetes. It is characterized by inadequate insulin secretion and resistance of peripheral tissues to insulin (Dc Fronzo, 1983). Patients with this type of diabetes are generally obese and obesity itself causes some degree of insulin resistance. Non-insulin dependent diabetes mellitus may result due to production of abnormal, biologically less active insulin molecule due to insulin gene mutation (Shoelson *et al.*, 1983). Non-insulin dependent diabetes mellitus patients do not require insulin for prevention for ketonuria and are not prone to ketosis. Due to insulin resistance, the blood glucose levels may be raised even in the presence of normal insulin levels, mild insulinopenia or higher insulin levels than the normal. Due to gradual development of hyperglycemia, this form of diabetes may remain undiagnosed for several years. Macrovascular and microvascular complications development risk increases in such patients. The risk factors involved in the development of NIDDM are age, obesity, lack of physical activity, urbanization and genetic susceptibility. Long term NIDDM increases the risks of complications such as retinopathy, nephropathy and neuropathy (Piero, 2006).

1.4.3   Gestational diabetes mellitus

Gestational diabetes refers to any degree of glucose intolerance with onset or primary identification during pregnancy usually in the second or third trimester (American Diabetes Association, 2001). Most of the cases of gestational diabetes resolve with delivery but fall in the risk category for the development of non-insulin dependent diabetes mellitus later in life (Sullivan, 1964). About 4% of all pregnancies are diagnosed with gestational diabetes. The indicators for the development of gestational diabetes are glycosuria, genetic predisposition, a past event of stillbirth or spontaneous abortion, incidence of malformation of the foetus in former pregnancy, a previous obese baby, maternal obesity, a high age of the mother and a parity of five or more. The timely recognition of GDM is important to prevent perinatal morbidity and mortality using effective therapy (Stowers and Sutherland, 1975).

1.4.4 Other specific types of diabetes

1.4.4.1 Diseases of the exocrine pancreas

The processes like pancreatitis, trauma infection, pancreatectomy and pancreatic carcinoma that cause severe injury to the pancreas can lead to the development of diabetes (American Diabetes Association, 2001). The extensive damage leads to destruction of β-cells by cystic fibrosis and hemochromatosis and impair insulin secretion. X-ray examination reveals fibrocalculous pancreatopathy associated with abdominal pain radiating to the back and pancreatic calcifications.

1.4.4.2 Endocrinopathies

Hormones such as growth hormone, cortisol, glucagon and epinephrine antagonize the action of insulin (American Diabetes Association, 2001). Excess of these hormones lead to conditions like acromegaly, Cushing's syndrome, glucagonoma and pheochromocytoma respectively which may result in the development of diabetes. The resultant hyperglycemia is usually rectified when the hormone excess is resolved.

1.4.4.3 Drug or chemical induced diabetes

Certain drugs which can hamper insulin secretion lead to the development of drug or chemical induced diabetes (Pandit *et al.,* 1993). This form of diabetes is generally precipitated in individuals with existing insulin resistance. Permanent destruction of β-cells occurs due to certain toxic substances like Vacor (a rat poison) and intravenous pentamidine (Assan *et al.,* 1995; Gallanosa *et al.,* 1981). Some of the drugs that induce diabetes are glucocorticoids, niacin, thiazides, dilantin and α-interferon (Yajnik *et al.,* 1995; Phelps *et al.,* 1989).

1.4.4.4 Genetic defects

Genetically determined abnormalities of insulin action can also cause diabetes (Rafel *et al.,* 1997). The mutations of insulin receptor lead to metabolic abnormalities ranging from hyperinsulinemia and modest hyperglycemia to severe diabetes. Monogenetic defects of β-cell function can also precipitate diabetes. In this form of diabetes, hyperglycemia occurs generally before 25 years of age and therefore referred to as the maturity onset diabetes of the young (MODY). Impaired insulin secretion with negligible or no defects in insulin action characterize this type of diabetes. These genetic defects are generally inherited in an autosomal dominant pattern.

1.5   Biochemical Background of Diabetes Mellitus

In the human body, every cell requires a regular source of energy for normal functioning. The primary energy source of the body cells is glucose, which circulates in the blood as mobilizable fuel source (Piero, 2006; Kibiti, 2006; Njagi, 2006). The regulation of glucose levels in the blood is carried out by a pancreatic hormone, insulin. Insulin binds to its specific receptor site on the plasma membrane and facilitates the entry of glucose into respiring cells and tissues. Conversion of glucose into pyruvate by glycolysis is stimulated by insulin. Excessive cytosolic glucose undergoes glycogenesis and excessive acetyl-CoA (acetyl coenzyme A) undergoes lipogenesis in the influence of insulin. Glucose starts staying in the blood rather than entering the cells, when the glucose levels are at or below threshold (Belinda, 2004).

In the hyperglycemic conditions, the water is drawn out of the cells into the blood stream and the excess sugar is excreted in the urine leading to the development of glycosuria (Piero, 2006) and the presentation of polydipsia and polyuria in the diabetic patients. Lack of insulin and prolong hyperglycemia result in lesser availability of glucose to the cells which start seeking alternative sources of energy such as fats, but fats are not the fuel sources for the red blood cells, kidney cortex and the brain. Blood brain barrier does not allow fatty acids to pass through. Catabolism of fatty acids generates acetyl-CoA which is diverted to ketogenesis to produce ketone bodies, which acts as an alternative fuel for such cells and tissues. The passage of these ketone bodies in urine lead to the development of ketonuria, which is a characteristic feature of diabetes mellitus. Ketosis results from the accumulation of ketone bodies in the blood and due to their acidic nature, lowers the pH of blood leading to acidosis. Ketoacidosis is a condition resulting from the combination of ketosis and acidosis and if not treated timely, may result in coma and death (Belinda, 2004).

1.6   Role of Insulin in Diabetes Mellitus

The β-cells of the islets of Langerhans in the pancreas synthesize a polypeptide hormone called insulin. The physiological functions of insulin on metabolism of carbohydrates include activation of transportation of glucose across muscle and adipocyte cell membranes, hepatic glycogen production regulation and suppression of glycogenolysis and gluconeogenesis resulting in lowering of blood glucose levels (Piero, 2006). The initiation of insulin action results after its binding to the specific receptor on the plasma membrane. Insulin carries out its enzymatic processes without entering the cell, with the help of second messenger that carries its signal to the interior of the cell (Kibiti, 2006). Insulin mediates tissue glucose uptake, maintains glucose homeostasis and clear the postprandial glucose load (Ginsberg, 1975; Reaven, 1983). The production of insulin is entirely dependent on the amount of sugar consumed. Deficiency of insulin plays an important role in the development of all forms of diabetes. As it is the primary hormone responsible for the uptake of glucose from the blood stream its deficiency to improper handling of glucose by body cells and improper storage of glucose in the liver and muscles. This eventually leads to perseveringly high blood glucose levels, poor protein synthesis and metabolic aberrations (WHO, 1999).

Insulin maintains blood glucose levels by regulating hepatic gluconeogenesis and promoting catabolism of glucose by skeletal muscles. In type-2 diabetes mellitus, the production of postabsorptive hepatic glucose increases which is directly related to the fasting plasma glucose concentration. Amongst gluconeogenesis and glycogenolysis, gluconeogenesis is remarkably increased in type-2 diabetes mellitus (Consoli, 1992). The persistent hyperglycemia emerging from diabetes mellitus, follows long term damage, dysfunction, and failure of organs like the eyes, kidneys, nerves, heart and blood vessels. Uncontrolled diabetes also accompanies hypertension and abnormalities of lipoprotein metabolism (Eren, 2004).

1.7   Structure of the Human Hand

The hand is one of the most interesting and highly developed biological motor systems. An inexhaustible number of activities, ranging from very simple to quite complex tasks are accomplished by our hand with the use of multiple digits simultaneously in a grasp or with the use of particular movements of individual units. Not only is the hand extremely useful and versatile, it is also quite complex.

1.7.1 The hand complex

The hand is the distal end of the upper extremity. It is composed of the thumb and four fingers. The hand complex comprises of a carpometacarpal joint and a metacarpophalangeal joint for each digit and two interphalangeal joints, the proximal and the distal for each finger. The thumb has only one interphalangeal joint. The proximal end of the metacarpals and phalanges is called the base, and the distal end is called the head (Chaurasia, 2004).

1.7.2 Joints and ligaments

1.7.2.1 Carpometacarpal joints

The joint between the trapezium and the base of the first metacarpal forms the carpometacarpal joint of the thumb. It is a saddle shaped joint which allows movement in two directions: abduction-adduction and opposition-reposition. The joint capsule is lax, which allows free movement but the range is controlled by strong ligaments.

The joints between the distal row of carpal bones and the second to fifth metacarpal bones are referred to as carpometacarpal joints of the fingers. These joints are hardly mobile, besides the joint with the fifth metacarpal, which allows modest movement in a palmar direction required for the opposition of the fifth finger. The dorsal and palmar carpometacarpal ligaments are provided to these joints, the fibers of which are in line with the axis of the metacarpal bones (Nakamura *et al.*, 2001). The bones are tied together with the intercarpal ligaments.

1.7.2.2 Metacarpophalangeal joints

The joint between the head of the first metacarpal and the base of its proximal phalanx forms the metacarpophalangeal joint of the thumb. It is different from that of the four fingers. Only flexion movement is allowed at this hinge joint (80-90°) and some extension in hypermobile individuals. In the palmar part of the capsule, two seasamoid bones are usually embedded.

The joint between convex metacarpal head proximally and the concave base of the first phalanx distally comprise the metacarpal joints of the fingers. In each of the second to fifth finger, the metacarpophalangeal joint is a ball and socket joint with a slack joint capsule, which is supported by strong palmar and collateral ligaments. The feasible movements are flexion (90°), extension (ocassionaly to 90°) and abduction-adduction, with index finger having highest mobility. (Chaurasia, 2004).

1.7.2.3 Interphalangeal joints

The joint between the head of the proximal phalanx and the base of the distal phalanx form the interphalangeal joint of the thumb which is structurally and functionally similar to the interphalangeal joints of the fingers, but unlike fingers, it lacks intermediate phalanx.

The head of proximal phalanx and the base of the intermediate phalanx comprise the proximal inerphalangeal joint and the head of the intermediate phalanx and the base of the distal phalanx form distal interphalangeal joint of each finger. These interphalangeal joints are hinges which allow flexion without extension. The range of flexion is more than 90° in the proximal interphalangeal joints which increases to 135° from the index to little finger and allows the formation of fist. In the distal interphalangeal joints, the range of flexion varies between 80° and 90° with highest mobility in little finger (Chaurasia, 2004).

1.7.3 Muscles and tendons

There are two types of muscles and tendons in the wrist, thumb and fingers-

a) Extrinsic muscles.

b) Intrinsic muscles.

1.7.3.1 Extrinsic muscles and tendons (Dorsal aspect)

Six osteofibrous tunnels can be distinguished on the dorsal aspect of the wrist which comprise of the abductor of the thumb and wrist extensors tendon sheaths.

i) Tunnel 1

This contains the tendons of -

a) The abductor pollicis longus - causes abduction of the thumb.

b) The extensor pollicis brevis - causes extension of the thumb.

Collectively they form the radial border of the 'anatomical snuffbox'.

ii) Tunnel 2

This contains the tendons of -

a) The extensor carpi radialis longus - combines with extensor carpi ulnaris to perform dorsiflexion of wrist.

b) The extensor carpi radialis brevis - causes extension of wrist.

iii) Tunnel 3

The third tunnel contains the tendon of -

a) The extensor pollicis longus - causes extension of the thumb, wrist and abduction of the thumb. It forms the ulnar border of the anatomical snuffbox.

iv) Tunnel 4

It comprises of five different tendons, the tendon of the extensor indicis proprius and four tendons of the extensor digitorium.

a) The extensor indicis proprius - causes extension of the index finger.

b) The extensor digitorium - causes the extension of the fingers, particularly proximal phalanges.

v) Tunnel 5

This contains one tendon of -

a) The extensor digiti minimi - causes extension of the fingers.

vi) Tunnel 6

This contains the tendon of -

a) The extensor carpi ulnaris - causes strong ulnar deviation of the wrist and opposition of the abductor pollicis longus.

1.7.3.2 Extrinsic muscles and tendons (Palmar aspect)

The tendons of the flexors of the wrist and fingers lie on palmar side, which are enclosed by the carpal tunnel and the tunnel of Guyon.

i) The tendinous structures enclosed within the carpal tunnel are -

   a) The flexor carpi radialis - flexes the wrist and helps in radial deviation.

   b) The palmaris longus - causes palmar flexion of the wrist and tenses the palmar fascia.

   c) The tendons of the superficial flexors of the fingers - causes flexion of the proximal phalanges of the fingers.

   d) The flexor carpi ulnaris - flexes the wrist.

   e) The flexor pollicis longus - flexes the thumb.

ii) The tunnel of Guyon is enclosed within the pisiform and hamate bone and is covered by the pisohamate ligament.

1.7.3.3 Intrinsic muscles

The intrinsic muscles of the hand are -

   a) The thenar muscle - include the abductor pollicis brevis, opponens pollicis and superficial and deeper head of flexor pollicis brevis and transverse and oblique head of adductor pollicis.

   b) The hypothenar muscles - include abductor digiti minimi, flexor digiti minimi brevis and opponens digiti minimi.

   c) The lumbrical muscles - consists of four lumbrical muscles which originate at the radial side of the tendons of the deep flexor digitorium muscle and insert at the dorsal aponeurosis of the fingers and at the joint capsules of metacarpophalangeal joints. They cause the flexion of metacarpophalangeal joints and extension of the interphalangeal joints.

   d) The palmar interossei - there are three palmar interossei which adduct the fingers in the direction of the middle finger. They cause the flexion of metacarpophalangeal joints and extension of interphalangeal joints of the fingers.

11

1.7.4 The dorsal interossei

The four dorsal interossei are very important. Each dorsal interossei has two heads, each in the side of the two adjacent metacarpal bones and originate from the sides of the five metacarpal bones. They attach into the extensor aponeurosis of the fingers as they move towards the proximal phalanges. Radial aspect of the index finger contains the first dorsal interosseus, the radial aspect of the middle finger contains the second dorsal interosseus, the third goes to the ulnar aspect of the middle finger and the fourth to the ulnar aspect of the fourth finger. The important function of the dorsal interossei is the abduction of the fingers away from the middle finger. They also cause the flexion of the metacarpophalangeal joints and extension of the interphalangeal joints.

1.7.5 The palmar aponeurosis

The continuation of the flexor retinaculum, which consists of the transverse and longitudinal fibers form the palmar aponeurosis of the hand. The transverse and longitudinal fibers of palmar aponeurosis are part of the tendon sheaths of the flexor tendons which also attach to the capsules of the metacarpophalangeal joints. It is also attached to the deep fascia of the hand, which is linked to its skeleton. The palmar aponeurosis forms a functional unit in conjuction with the ligaments, septa and fasciae. It protects the soft tissues of the mid-hand during a strong grip by fixing the skin of the palm to the metacarpal bones.

1.8 Biomechanics of the Human Hand

1.8.1 Range of motion of the human hand

The range of motion in each joint of the human hand has been approximately delimited after an extensive research using specialized equipment, as shown in the following table 1.2 :

Table 1.2: Range of motion in finger joints (cited from Cobos *et al.*, 2008)

Finger	Flexion	Extension	Abduction/adduction
Thumb			
Trapeziometacarpal	50°-90°	15°	45°-60°
Metacarpophalangeal	75°-80°	0°	0°
Interphalangeal	75°-80°	5°-10°	0°
Index Finger			
Carpometacarpal	5°	0°	0°
Metacarpophalangeal	90°	30°-40°	60°
Proximal interphalangeal	110°	0°	0°
Distal interphalangeal	80-90^0	5°	0°
Middle Finger			
Carpometacarpal	5°	0°	0°
Metacarpophalangeal	90°	30°-40°	45°
Proximal interphalangeal	110°	0°	0°
Distal interphalangeal	80-90^0	5°	0°
Ring Finger			
Carpometacarpal	10°	0°	0°
Metacarpophalangeal	90°	30°-40°	45°
Proximal interphalangeal	120°	0°	0°
Distal interphalangeal	80-90^0	5°	0°
Little Finger			
Carpometacarpal	15°	0°	0°
Metacarpophalangeal	90°	30°-40°	50°
Proximal interphalangeal	135°	0°	0°
Distal interphalangeal	90^0	5°	0°

Table 1.3: Range of motion in the wrist (cited from Marshall *et al.*, 1999)

Wrist	Value
Flexion	$65°-70°$
Extension	$70°-80°$
Radial flexion (deviation)	$15°-25°$
Ulnar flexion (deviation)	$40°-45°$

1.8.2 Types of grasp

The hand is able to grasp or hold an object between any two surfaces of hand with the help of prehensile activities. In context of biomechanical motion, the hand possesses seven movements that make up maximum of the hand functions.

i) The precision pinch - It is also known as the terminal pinch. Flexion of the interphalangeal joint of the thumb and the distal interphalangeal joint of the index finger is involved in the precision pinch. It helps in picking up of small items such as a pen by bringing together the tips of the fingernails.

ii) The oppositional pinch - It is also known as the subterminal pinch. It involves the extension of interphalangeal joints and distal interphalangeal joints by bringing together the pulp of the thumb and index finger. The contraction of the first dorsal interosseous, together with the flexion of the index profundus is also involved.

iii) The key pinch - It involves the adduction of the thumb to the radial aspect of the index finger's middle phalanx. The index finger is the stable pillar of this type of movement. It requires sufficient length of the digit and a metacarpal phalangeal joint, efficient to resist the adduction of the thumb.

iv) The chuck grip - It is also known as the directional grip. With this type of grip, the hand is able to hold a cylindrical object involving the index finger, middle finger and thumb. In this type of grip, a rotational and axial force is generally applied to the object.

v) The hook grip - Flexion of the finger at the interphalangeal joint and metacarpophalangeal joint extension is required in this type of grip. The picking up of a suitcase or briefcase, which does not require thumb action utilize this type of grip.

vi) The power grasp - This type of grip involves flexion of fingers and thumb which are opposed relative to the other digits, for example, gripping a club or bat.

vii) The span grasp - This type of grip involves generation of the forces between the thumb and fingers with the help of flexion of distal interphalangeal joints and the proximal interphalangeal joints to around $30°$ and the palmar abduction of the thumb. The thumb, metacarpophalangeal and interphalangeal joints stabnility is required, for example to grab a ball.

1.9 Handgrip Strength

The highest voluntary force that an individual can wield under normal biokinetic conditions, resulting from the forceful flexion of all finger joints, thumb and wrist depicts the strength of a handgrip (Koley and Yadav, 2009). Grip strength is the combined activity of muscles that can be executed in one single muscular contraction (Nwuga, 1975). To assess the functional integrity of the hand as the part of the musculoskeletal system, grip strength is a reliable and authentic measure (Rhind *et al.*, 1980). Grip strength is a reliable and valid evaluation of hand strength and can provide an objective index of hand and upper body strength (Methot *et al.*, 2010) Handgrip strength is an indicator of numerous physiological systems, its increment may be a beneficial approach to enhance general health and lower the chances of occurrence of multiple chronic diseases and premature mortality (Cheung *et al.*, 2013). It is evaluated by calculating the extent of static force that the hand is able to generate while compressing a dynamometer. In the clinical settings, grip strength is also evaluated as a marker of disease activity (Rhind *et al.*, 1980). The estimation of handgrip strength bears a great significance in the determination of upper limb damage, measurement of decrement in hand muscle power, treatment goal setting, rehabilitation progress monitoring and assessing capability of patients to return to employment (Blair *et al.*, 1987; Mathiowetz *et al.*, 1984).

Handgrip strength being a physiological variable, is affected by numerous parameters including age, gender, body size among many others. Previous researches by Benefice and Malina *et al.* (1996) and Hager-Ross and Rosblad (2002) have established strong correlations between grip strength and a number of anthropometric traits. With advancing age, decline in handgrip strength is observed in both males and females (Kamarul *et al.*, 2006). In a study conducted by Mathiowetz *et al.* (1985), the highest values of grip strength were recorded for the age group between 25 to 39 years and a gradual decline is observed in the age group of 60 to 79 years. Greater muscle mass and larger amount of contractile tissue in males lead to greater grip strength in males as compared to females (Shetty *et al.*, 2012). Grip strength is found to be higher in the dominant hand in the right handed people as compared to the non-dominant hand but in case of the left handed people, no such differences could be observed (Incel *et al.*, 2002). As suggested by Chatterjee and Chowdhuri (1991), handgrip strength showed positive correlation with weight, height and body surface area. Handgrip strength is a remarkable indicator of bone mineral content and bone area at the forearm sites and positively correlated with lean body mass and physical activity (Karkkainen *et al.*, 2009). Handgrip strength also shows powerful correlation with hip/waist circumferences as they indicate the distribution of fat in the body (Brozek, 1984). Hand size must be taken into consideration while measuring handgrip strength (Jonathan *et al.*, 2002). Maximum grip strength also possesses strong correlation with hand circumference in both males and females (Hemberal *et al.*, 2014).

The assessment of grip strength is important in determining the overall muscle strength of the body (Bassey and Harries, 1993; Koley *et al.*, 2009). It may be helpful in the diagnosis and follow-up of neuromuscular disease patients (Wiles *et al.*, 1990). Handgrip strength determines the efficacy of various treatment strategies of hand and also in hand rehabilitation. Handgrip strength can also be used as functional index of nutritional status (Brozek, 1984; JeeJeebhoy, 1998; Vaz *et al.*, 1996; Guo *et al.*, 1996).

1.9.1 Handgrip strength and type-2 diabetes mellitus

Individuals with longstanding type-2 diabetic patients experience limitations of upper limb function and physical disability (Ozdirenc *et al.*, 2003; Clerke and

Clerke, 2001). The chronic complications that occur in diabetic patients decrease their quality of life. In diabetic individuals, the hand is an organ system that is primarily damaged, which is accompanied by impaired function and discomfort for the patients. Handgrip strength has been particularly seen to be related to overall fitness in individuals with diabetes mellitus and as an established marker for conditioning (Wallymahmed *et al.*, 2007). In old age people, the decrement in muscle mass and strength with advancing age is significantly associated with type-2 diabetes mellitus (Centinus *et al.*, 2005; Sayer *et al.*, 2005). Due to loss of muscle strength, reduced handgrip strength is observed along with the development of physical disability in diabetes (Eves and Plotnikoff, 2006; Kondo *et al.*, 2006). The development of physical disabilities in diabetic individuals makes them more disabled in self care tasks as compared to normal age matched individuals. Higher reduction of handgrip strength and agility is seen with increase in duration of type-2 diabetes (Savas *et al.*, 2007; Gamstedt *et al.*, 1993). Association of the duration of diabetes of more than 6 years and poor glycemic control with reduced muscle quality and higher prevalence of musculoskeletal conditions like carpel-tunnel syndrome, muscle atrophy and Duputyren's contracture was observed by Deal (1998).

Decline in muscle strength with type-2 diabetes mellitus is observed in both males and females (Centinus *et al.*, 2005). According to Goopaster *et al.* (2006), Hurley (1995) and Sinaki *et al.* (2001), men experience more rapid decline in muscle strength, mass and quality as compared to women with aging. In older males elevated fasting glucose levels are found to be more common than older females, but elevated postchallenge glucose levels in older females as compared to older males. Study by Park *et al.* (2006) suggested that males suffering from diabetes have lower appendicular muscle strength regardless of greater appendicular muscle mass, in comparison to non-diabetic males, but no such association was reported in females. Dysglycemia poses as a risk factor for decline in grip strength, an indicator for overall reduced muscle strength, especially in men and finally to the augmentation of functional limitations and physical impairments in older adults (Kalyani *et al.*, 2015). However, lesser attention has been paid to functioning of hand in type-2 diabetic patients as compared to diabetic foot and other diabetic complications (Redmond *et al.*, 2009). To fill the void of literature related to the strength of hand in patients with type-2 diabetes mellitus, especially in north Indian context, the present study was planned.

1.10   Aims and Objectives

The aims of the present study were:

- To estimate the handgrip strength of patients with type-2 diabetes mellitus.

- To estimate the handgrip strength of age, sex matched controls.

- To compare the handgrip strength between the patients with type-2 diabetes mellitus and controls.

- To estimate the sex differences for handgrip strength in patients with type-2 diabetes mellitus and controls.

- To establish correlations with handgrip strength and selected anthropometric measurements in patients with type-2 diabetes mellitus.

1.11   Hypothesis

There would be significant differences in handgrip strength between patients with type-2 diabetes mellitus and controls age group-wise. There would be significant correlations between handgrip strength and selected anthropometric variables in patients with type-2 diabetes mellitus.

REVIEW OF LITERATURE

A review of literature is a body of text that aims to review the critical points of current knowledge. It comprises of particular field of research based comprehensive survey of publications. Reviewing the literature provides information on the conclusions and interpretations of the previous research findings. It is a process of documenting the particular topic related current relevant research literature. In order to conduct any scientific study, the review of previous studies done on the topic is preliminary requirement, as it avoids duplication of the study, adds up new ideas and helps in verification of the theories and making hypothesis.

In the present study, the literature for the review was collected from Bhai Gurdas Library, Guru Nanak Dev University, Amritsar and from electronic media sites like www.google.com, www.scihub.com, www.pubmed.com and www.sciencedirect.com.

2.1 Handgrip Strength in Patients with Type-2 Diabetes Mellitus

Akpinar *et al.* (2017) carried observational case control study to assess the functioning of hand in type 2 diabetic patients. The participants of the study consisted of ninety-one type-2 diabetic patients aged 40-65 years and sixty age and sex matched non-diabetic controls. Functional hand disability was measured by Duruoz Hand Index. Handgrip strength was measured by Jamar dynamometer. In patients with type-2, diabetes mellitus significantly higher scores of Duruoz Hand Index were observed as compared to scores in non-diabetic subjects. In type-2 diabetic patients and controls, no significant differences were observed in their handgrip values. However, grip strength and Duruoz Hand Index scores had negatively significant correlation in type-2 diabetic subjects.

Ibrahim (2016) studied the effect of type-2 diabetes mellitus on handgrip strength in young males of Hail City-KSA. The subjects were divided into two groups ie., Group A and Group B. Group A consisted of 15 diabetic subjects and Group B consisted of 15 non-diabetic subjects. Handgrip strength was measured using Jamar hydraulic hand dynamometer and pinch strength with pinch gauge. Significant reduction of handgrip strength in both right and left hand was noted in diabetic subjects as compared to non-diabetic subjects. Right and left thumb strength in the diabetic group was also significantly lower in diabetic males as compared to normal males. The study established the importance of handgrip strength and thumb strength as important parameters of hand function which were significantly affected by diabetes, leading to the development of hand disabilities.

Gill *et al.* (2016) conducted a cross sectional study on handgrip strength in type-2 diabetic males. The study involved fifty type-2 diabetic males in the age group of 50-60 years with duration of diabetes of more than 10 years, and fifty age and sex matched controls. The handgrip strength was measured using Jamar hand held dynamometer. Significantly lower mean values of handgrip strength were observed in diabetic patients as compared to control counterparts, where as significantly higher mean values of weight and body mass index were reported in diabetic patients as compared to controls. They explained the decrease in strength of muscles in diabetic individuals as compared to healthy age matched controls, due to increased resistance of tissues to insulin and hyperglycaemia which resulted in decreased number of mitochondria in the muscle cells and reduced synthesis of glycogen.

Al Shreef *et al.* (2015) examined the effect of aerobic and resistance training on bone metabolism and handgrip strength in 100 non-insulin dependent type-2 diabetic male patients from Saudi Arabia divided into two subgroups - Group A and Group B. Group A patients received aerobic training session on a treadmill at a low load for 30 minutes. The beginning of the session included a 10 minute stretching session. For first two weeks session was performed at 60-70% of HR max and third to twelfth weeks at 70-80% of HR max. Group B patients were subjected to 40 minute resistance training session on eight resistance machines-chest press, biceps curl, triceps extension, lower back, abdominals, leg press, leg curl and leg extension. The participants carried out three sets of 8-12 repetitions with 60 seconds of rest between each set. The comparison between the groups was done using independent t-test. The training sessions continued for 6 months. Handgrip strength, parathyroid hormone and calcium levels were measured before and the end of training session. Significant differences were observed in values of handgrip strength, parathyroid hormone and calcium levels in both groups before and after the training sessions. Significantly higher improvements in values of handgrip strength and calcium levels were recorded for group A receiving aerobic training. The study referred the aerobic training as the effective method to improve bone metabolism markers and handgrip strength in non-insulin dependent type-2 diabetic patients.

Amaral *et al.* (2015) conducted a population based study on 1395 adult males and females of Rio Branco, Acre State and Brazil to analyze the association of handgrip strength and self reported diseases and multi morbidity. Handgrip strength was measured using hydraulic hand held dynamometer. In men, handgrip strength was significantly higher as compared to women. The results also revealed that men with lower handgrip strength were more likely to have hypertension, diabetes, musculoskeletal disorders, and multi morbidity after controlling for age group, body mass index and physical activity. In the multivariate models associations between handgrip strength and cardiovascular disease, dyslipidemia, musculoskeletal disorders and multimorbidity amongst women were not sustained. The use of handgrip strength as a health biomarker was suggested by the study.

Shambhuvani *et al.* (2015) conducted an observational study on 25 subjects with type-2 diabetes mellitus diagnosed since more than 6 years and aged between 35-75 years. The handgrip strength of the diabetic subjects was measured using Jamar hydraulic hand-held dynamometer. The results were compared with 25 apparently healthy age-matched non-diabetic subjects. They illustrated that handgrip strength of subjects with long standing type-2 diabetes mellitus was considerably lower than non-diabetic individuals. Significant difference was also observed between the handgrip strength of dominant and non-dominant hand in diabetic and healthy subjects. They attributed the decline of handgrip strength in diabetic subjects to increased insulin tissue resistance and hyperglycaemia and also to the lower physiological cross section of the muscles which worsen with increased duration and improper control of diabetes.

Van-Der-Kooi *et al.* (2015) explored the relation of type-2 diabetes and handgrip strength in six ethnic groups from the HELIUS study (Healthy life in an urban setting study). The study sample included 2086 Dutch, 2216 South Asian Surinamese, 2084 African Surinamese, 1786 Ghanaian, 2223 Turkish and 2199 Moroccan origin type-2 diabetic individuals on either diabetic medication or with fasting glucose level of ≥7.0 m mol/L and controls without diabetes. Citec hand-held dynamometer was used to measure handgrip strength. Body measurements of height, body weight, hip circumference and waist circumference were also recorded. The relation between handgrip strength and type-2 diabetes mellitus was analyzed using logistic regression. The results showed variation in body composition among ethnic groups. The highest values of body mass index and waist circumference were observed in Turkish subjects and percent body fat in Moroccan subjects, while the lowest values for all the variables were found in Dutch participants. Higher mean values of handgrip strength were recorded for men as compared to women. Handgrip strength was found to be higher in the subjects without type-2 diabetes mellitus in comparison to subjects with type-2 diabetes mellitus in all the ethnic groups. Significant differences of handgrip strength (p≤ 0.001) were observed between the ethnic groups. For both men and women, greater values for handgrip strength among all the ethnic groups were observed in Dutch whereas least values of handgrip strength were seen in South Asian Surinamese men and women.

Abdel Fattah *et al.* (2014) studied the association between nerve conduction velocity and handgrip strength in non-insulin dependent type-2 diabetic individuals. The study included 30 type-2 diabetic male patients age ranging from 45 to 55 years and with BMI within the range of 25-29.9 kg/m^2 along with thirty age and sex matched healthy controls. Handgrip strength of both groups was measured using hydraulic hand dynamometer in a seated position. Nerve conduction velocity of median nerve of dominant hand of both groups was recorded using standard electromyographic equipment. The correlation between handgrip strength and nerve conduction velocity in the diabetic group was calculated using Pearson's correlation coefficient. The mean scores of handgrip strength in the diabetic group were significantly lower than the control group. Statistically significant reduction (p≤0.001) of mean values of nerve conduction velocity were observed in the diabetic group. The duration of diabetes showed significant negative correlation with both handgrip strength and nerve conduction velocity.

Khallaf *et al.* (2014) conducted a cross-sectional study in the outpatient clinics of King Khalid Hospital measuring the long duration effects of type-2 diabetes mellitus on handgrip strength and pinch power of females in the city of Hail-KSA.

22

The study involved 40 female diabetic subjects (mean age 51±5.58 years) with mean duration of illness of 7.8±1.46 years, and 40 healthy age and sex matched controls with no glucose intolerance, pain history or musculoskeletal problem in the shoulder or hand. Majority of the participants were right hand dominant. The measurements of body weight were taken using a calibrated scale and handgrip strength and key pinch power were taken using Jamar hydraulic dynamometer in a seated position with shoulder adducted and neutrally rotated, elbow flexed at 90° and neutral position of forearm and wrist. The maximum reading was recorded. In results, significantly lower values ($p \leq 0.005$) of handgrip strength and key pinch power were observed for diabetic females both in right and left hand as compared to the control group. The study concluded that long standing type-2 diabetes mellitus increased the risk of development of functional disabilities due to weakness of muscles of hand.

Cheung *et al.* (2013) carried out a cross-sectional cohort study to assess the relationship of handgrip strength with chronic diseases and multi morbidity. The data was collected from Southern Chinese 748 men and 397 women aged 50 years from 1998 to 2009. For the study, 18 chronic diseases including diabetes were selected which were prevalent in $\geq 1\%$ of the population. Handgrip strength was measured using Smedley hand dynamometer. The study revealed that decreased handgrip strength in men was associated with increased odds of 12 chronic diseases and in women with 8 chronic diseases including diabetes. The results of multivariable ANCOVA (analysis of covariance) analysis depicted a significant positive linear relationship between age and number of chronic diseases in women but not in men. Significant negative linear relation between handgrip strength and number of chronic diseases was observed for men but not in women.

Leenders *et al.* (2013) demonstrated a larger descent in muscle mass, muscle strength and functional capacity in patients with type-2 diabetes mellitus with aging. The study involved 60 type-2 diabetic males aged above 70 years and 32 sex and age matched controls with normal glycemic levels. Dual energy x-ray absorptiometry (DEXA) was used to measure body composition and bone mineral content. 1-repetition maximum (1RM) strength tests on leg press and leg extension machines assessed maximum strength. Sit to stand test and handgrip test were used as measures of physical performance. For body mass and fat mass, no significant

23

differences were observed between normal subjects and type-2 diabetic subjects. Significantly lower values of leg extension strength were observed for type-2 diabetic individuals. Type-2 diabetic individuals observed significantly longer sit to stand time and significantly lower values of handgrip strength as compared to non-diabetic subjects.

Siddiqui *et al.* (2013) reported the differences among diabetic and non-diabetic individuals for two point discrimination and grip strength. The study recruited 30 type-2 diabetic males and females with mean age of 48.03±6.0 years and 30 age and sex matched controls. The grip strength was measured by Jamar hand dynamometer. The measurement of two point discrimination for dominant hand was done using aesthesiometer. The sensations were checked in the dermatomes C_6 (thumb), C_7 (middle finger) and C_8 (little finger). Significantly lower mean values of handgrip strength were observed for diabetic individuals as compared to controls. Significant differences in two point discrimination in C_7 were observed among diabetic and non-diabetic individuals, whereas for dermatome of C_8 no significant difference was observed. The study indicated the importance of evaluation of sensibility in the hand of the type-2 diabetic patients, to timely evaluate the extent of the sensory changes and upper limb neuropathy.

Sindhur *et al.* (2013) carried out a comparative study to determine the handgrip strength in type-2 diabetic and non-diabetic subjects. The study comprised of 274 subjects (137 diabetic and 137 normal individuals). Hand dynamometer was used to measure handgrip strength. Significant reduction of grip strength was observed in diabetic individuals. In diabetic individuals, the decline in grip strength becames more pronounced with increase in age. The study concluded that reduction in muscular strength as indicated by grip strength decline was contributed by poor glycemic control with raised systemic inflammatory cytokines and interleukin which had damaging effect on muscle function.

Andersen (2012) presented a review article on motor dysfunction in diabetic patients. Decreased muscle strength was found at the knee and at the ankle in type-1 and type-2 diabetic patients. In diabetic patients with polyneuropathy, muscle weakness was observed while normal strength was noted in non-neuropathic patients even with long term diabetes. Signs and severity of polyneuropathy were found closely related to muscle weakness. Lower muscle quality was recorded for diabetic patients, which further declined with longer duration of diabetes and poor glycemic control. Grip strength according to a cross sectional survey of 1400 diabetic subjects, was lower in diabetic patients as well in patients with impaired glucose tolerance. Muscle atrophy was diagnosed in parallel with muscle weakness in patients with diabetic neuropathy. Foot ulcer development risk was increased due to muscle atrophy induced alterations of the biomechanics of the foot. It was concluded that strength, postural stability, and walking performance can be improved by muscle and balance training.

Ezema *et al.* (2012) studied the effect of long standing type-2 diabetes mellitus on handgrip strength. The study involved the participation of 40 individuals which were divided into two groups. Group A consisted of 20 non-diabetic subjects (10 males and 10 females) and group B consisted of type-2 diabetic patients with duration of diabetes of more than 6 years (10 males and 10 females). The participants were all right handed and aged between 39-65 years. The handgrip was measured using Saehan hydraulic dynamometer. Significant differences were observed in handgrip strength of diabetic and non-diabetic males ($p \leq 0.004$) and diabetic and non-diabetic females ($p \leq 0.002$). The study clearly revealed that muscle quality of upper limb was consistently lower in both male and female type-2 diabetic patients with long duration of diabetes (>6 years).

Shah *et al.* (2011) conducted a cross sectional study to evaluate handgrip strength and endurance in type-2 diabetic patients. The subjects comprised of 60 type-2 non-insulin dependent diabetic males aged 40-60 years and 60 normal, age and sex matched controls. The handgrip strength of the subjects was measured using handgrip dynamometer (INCO India ltd.). The handgrip endurance of the subjects was measured by the maximum duration for which they maintained the grip on the handgrip dynamometer at 1/3 of their maximum handgrip strength. Significant differences were observed for handgrip strength among diabetics and controls. Significantly lower mean values of handgrip strength were observed for diabetics as compared to normal controls. The diabetic group also exhibited significantly lower mean values of handgrip endurance as compared to controls.

Stenholm *et al.* (2011) carried a survey based study on 2021 men and women aged 55 years and above in Finland. They evaluated the relation between history of obesity and handgrip strength in elderly adults and investigated the role of inflammation and insulin resistance as mediating factors. The data obtained included body mass, body height, maximal handgrip strength, C-reactive protein and homeostasis model assessment (HOMA-IR) based insulin resistance. Hierarchical classification of obesity history was obtained by recalling weight at 20, 30, 40 and 50 years of age. Individuals with body mass index ≥ 30 kg/m^2 were considered to be obese. After controlling for age, sex, education, smoking, alcohol use, physical activity, several chronic diseases and current body weight earlier onset of obesity was related with lower handgrip strength. As compared with never obese participants adjusted logistic regression models depicted that odds for very low relative handgrip strength were 2.76 (1.78-4.28) for currently obese, 5.57 (3.02-10.28) for obese since age of 50 years, 6.53 (2.98-14.30) for obese since age of 40 years, and 10.36 (3.55-30.24) for obese since age of 30 years. Higher levels of CRP and HOMA-IR and early onset of obesity correlated with lower handgrip strength.

Wander *et al.* (2011) assessed handgrip strength as a possible predictor of incident diabetes. The study involved 394 non-diabetic lean Japanese-American individuals (mean age 51.9 years) followed for the development of diabetes at 10 years. A ten year follow assessment of the subjects was performed and compared with baseline measurements. Handgrip strength was measured using Harpenden dynamometer. The association between handgrip strength and odds of incident diabetes were estimated using logistic regression after adjusting for age, sex and family history. Handgrip strength and type-2 diabetes risk possessed statistically significant ($p \leq 0.008$) and negative (coefficient -0.208) association. With BMI set at 25th, 50th or 75th percentiles at adjusted odd ratios for a 10-pound handgrip strength increase were 0.68, 0.79 and 0.98 respectively. The study indicated greater handgrip strength was associated with decreased risk of developing type-2 diabetes among lean Japanese- American subjects.

Nomura *et al.* (2007) carried out a pilot study to establish muscle strength as a marker of insulin resistance in type-2 diabetic patients. The study recruited 20 male and 20 female type-2 diabetic subjects with mean age of 53.3 ±12.7 years. Subjects undergoing insulin therapy or antidiabetic drugs like thiazolidinediones and biguanides affecting insulin sensitivity were excluded from the study. Knee extensors maximal isometric muscle strength was measured using dynamometer. The values of fasting plasma glucose, HbA1c, serum insulin levels, total cholesterol, HDL-cholesterol and triglyceride concentrations were also recorded. Homeostatic Model Assessment (HOMA) was used to estimate the degree of insulin resistance. Significant correlation was observed between the knee extension force normalized for body weight (% KEF) and HOMA-IR in both male ($p \leq 0.05$) and female ($p \leq 0.05$) subjects. % KEF ($p \leq 0.005$) and BMI ($p \leq 0.05$) were evaluated as independent determinants of HOMA-IR. As lower extremity muscle strength was found to be independently associated with insulin resistance, the study confirmed the previous reports of glycemic control being improved by resistance training in type-2 diabetic subjects.

Sayer *et al.* (2007) established the association between age related loss of muscle mass and strength in old age type-2 diabetic patients. The study involved 2677 men and women aged 59-73 years. The data obtained included grip strength, fasting glucose, triglycerides and HDL cholesterol, blood pressure, waist circumference and 2h glucose levels. Significant association ($p \leq 0.001$) of grip strength was observed with weight, height and fat mass. In gender adjusted analysis, only high blood pressure, waist circumference and 2h glucose levels were associated with grip strength. Significant association of SD (standard deviation) decrease in grip strength was observed with fasting triglycerides ($p \leq 0.006$), blood pressure ($p \leq 0.004$), waist circumference ($p \leq 0.001$), 2h glucose ($p \leq 0.001$), and higher possibility of having the metabolic syndrome as per the ATPlll ($p \leq 0.001$) and IDF definitions ($p \leq 0.03$). The study evidenced that adverse metabolic profile impaired grip strength as a result of loss of physical function.

Park *et al.* (2006) studied the decrease in muscular strength and quality in elderly individuals with type-2 diabetes. Grip and knee extensor strength and muscle mass was evaluated in 485 type-2 diabetic and 2133 non-diabetic individuals in the health, aging and body composition study. Knee extension strength was measured using isokinetic dynamometer and grip strength was measured with Jamar dynamometer. Despite significantly greater arm and leg muscle mass ($p \leq 0.001$) in diabetic individuals, lower muscle strength in both upper and lower extremities (p≤0.05) in diabetic males was reported. No significant differences in absolute arm and leg muscle strength were observed in diabetic and non-diabetic females. In both men and women with diabetes, muscle quality was significantly lower (p≤0.001) in both upper and lower extremities as compared to non-diabetic individuals. Lowest muscle quality was observed in diabetic individuals with longer duration of diabetes (≥6 years) and with poor glycemic control (HbA1c>8.0%) regardless of sex and muscle groups examined. The study indicated the development of physical disability in elderly individuals with diabetes.

Centinus *et al.* (2005) assessed handgrip strength in patients with type-2 diabetes mellitus. The study was conducted at the department of Internal Medicine, Kahramanmaras Suctu Imam University, Turkey. The study included 76 patients with type-2 diabetes mellitus (mean age 50.11 ±7.6 years) diagnosed after glucose challenge test and 47 healthy subjects (mean age 46.93 ±10.2 years) with no glucose irregularities. Handgrip strength was measured using a calibrated Jamar dynamometer and pinch power with a pinch gauge. Significantly (p≤0.05) lower handgrip strength values were observed for the diabetic group. The key pinch power values were recorded to be significantly lower (p≤0.05) in diabetic individuals in the right hand. When classified according to age in both diabetic and control group, handgrip strength and pinch power values were found to be significantly lower in diabetic group in both 30-49 years and more than 50 years age groups. 34.9% of the diabetic patients reported that decreased hand power affected their daily activities.

Sayer *et al.* (2005) carried out a cross sectional study to evaluate the association among glucose tolerance, muscle strength and physical function in type-2 diabetic and non-diabetic males and females. The study sample included 1391 men and women living in the English county of Hertfordshire aged between 60 and 70 years. Grip strength was measured using Jamar dynamometer. Significantly reduced mean handgrip strength (p≤0.002) was observed in diabetic males as compared with males with impaired glucose tolerance and with males having normal glucose tolerance. SD rise in glucose concentration was associated with significant reduction in grip strength (p≤0.001) after adjustment for weight. In case of diabetic men, the odds ratio of reduced physical function as compared to males with normal glucose tolerance was 2.73 (p≤0.001) and males with impaired glucose tolerance with normal glucose levels (p≤0.03). The relationship between these variables was not clear in females.

Andersen *et al.* (2004) evaluated the effect of type-2 diabetes on strength of the muscles by measuring the strength of the flexors and extensors at elbow, wrist, knee and ankle in 36 type-2 diabetic subjects with diabetes duration of more than 5 years and 36 control subjects matched for sex, age, weight, height and physical activity. Clinical scores, nerve conduction studies and quantitative sensory testing were the determinants of degree of neuropathy. Neuropathy rank sum score (NRSS) was obtained after analysis of all the results. Retinal condition and extent of nephropathy was also evaluated. A significant reduction of strength by 17% of ankle flexors (p≤0.02) and 14% of ankle flexors (p≤0.03) was seen in diabetic patients. Strength of extensors and flexors at the knee was reduced by 7% and 14% (p≤0.05) respectively. Strength at the ankle (r =-0.45, p≤0.01) and the knee (r =-0.42, p≤0.02) was associated with NRSS. The results of multiple regression analysis associated NRSS with strength at the ankle and knee but not the degree of nephropathy and retinopathy.

2.2 Hand Disability in Patients with Type-2 Diabetes Mellitus

McGrath *et al.* (2017) analyzed the data from the longitudinal study Hispanic Established Population for the Epidemiological Study of the Elderly (HEPESE) to determine the effects of muscle weakness and type-2 diabetes mellitus on incident activities of daily living disability (ADL) in elderly Mexican Americans. The study followed subsample of 2270 Mexican Americans aged 65 years at baseline, for 19 years. Jamar hand-held dynamometer was used to assess handgrip strength. Normalized handgrip strength (NGS) was determined by normalizing handgrip strength to body weight. Male subjects with NGS values of ≤0.46 and females with NGS values of ≤0.30 were considered weak. The subjects that had diabetes only, were weak only, and were both weak and had diabetes had a 1.94 (CI= [1.89, 1.98]), 1.17 (CI= [1.16, 1.19]), 2.12 (CI= [2.08, 2.16]) higher rate for incident disability as compared to subjects that were not weak and did not had diabetes. The study

29

identified both muscle weakness and diabetes to be jointly and independently related with elevated rates for incident ADL disability in elderly Mexican Americans.

Lewko *et al.* (2012) studied the effects of diabetes related limited hand function on quality of life. The study included 21 type-1 diabetic patients and 50 type-2 diabetic patients aged under 80 years. The data on hand function and quality of life was collected using health related quality of life index (QLI), Acceptance of Illness Scale (AIS), Barthel Index, and the Hospital Anxiety and Depression Scale (HADS) questionnaire. Distal motor latency and conduction velocity was also measured. Median nerve neuropathy was diagnosed as distal latencies greater than 3.8 ms (milliseconds) and conduction velocities above 50 m/s (meters per second). Difficulty was experienced by patients to lift objects in the right ($p \leq 0.05$) and left hand ($p \leq 0.004$) with damaged distal latency. The quality of life in patients with limited hand functions was significantly lower than patients without any symptoms according to Quality of Life Index. Reduced hand function and quality of life had a significant negative effect on Acceptance of Illness Scale, the incidence of depressive symptoms ($p \leq 0.001$) and the patient's functional status.

Redmond *et al.* (2009) identified the disability patterns of various diabetic hand conditions and factors that resulted in reduced hand function. The participants involved 60 adults (26 males, 34 females) with type 1 or 2 diabetes with mean age of 60.9 ±10.5 years and with at least one of the following hand related disorders: carpel tunnel syndrome, trigger finger, Dupuytren's disease, or limited joint mobility syndrome. Hand disability and health status were measured using two questionnaires-The Disabilities of the Arm, Shoulder and Hand (DASH) and Medical Outcomes Study Short Form-36 (SF-36v2). Handgrip strength was measured using EVAL electrodynamometer, light touch perception by WEST hand set of monofilaments and finger dexterity by Rolyan 9-hole peg test. Carpel tunnel syndrome was the most frequently presented disorder (45%) but presentation of clinical features of more than one hand syndrome was also common (47%). Greater hand disability patterns were observed in females with significantly higher DASH scores than men ($p \leq 0.01$). Significant associations of hand disability were observed with grip strength, dexterity, and obesity ($p \leq 0.05$).

30

2.3 Hand Abnormalities in Patients with Type-2 Diabetes Mellitus

Gamstedt *et al.* (1993) carried out a cross sectional study on 100 diabetic patients to evaluate the prevalence of hand abnormalities and its relation with various variables, ergonomic factors, smoking habits and duration of diabetes. About 20% of the patients were diagnosed with carpal tunnel syndrome, Duputyren's contracture, flexor tenosynovitis and limited joint mobility each. Abnormalities of hand were seen in 50 patients and 26 patients had more than one abnormality and were associated with duration of diabetes. 18% of patients suffered from hand abnormalities with duration of diabetes of less than 10 years and 78% of those with 20 years or longer duration. An inverse relation was observed between risk of hand abnormalities and metabolic control. No significant relationship was observed between hand abnormalities and smoking habits. Out of 50 patients, 25 were disabled to such an extent that surgery was recommended.

Jennings *et al.* (1989) assessed 233 type-2 diabetic patients for complications like limited finger joint mobility and Duputyren's contracture. About 26 % of the subjects were diagnosed with Duputyren's contracture and 34% with limited joint mobility. With increased duration of diabetes and age, there was increased incidence of limited joint mobility and Duputyren's contracture. The logistic regression analysis presented significant association of limited joint mobility with retinopathy and Duputyren's contracture and independent association of Duputyren's contracture with vision-threatening retinopathy limited joint mobility and foot ulceration after adjusting for age and limited joint mobility. The study surfaced the fact that diabetes may lead to connective tissue abnormalities which further lead to a number of diabetic complications.

Starkman *et al.* (1986) studied the association of limited joint mobility (LJM) and its complications with diabetes mellitus. The study involved 361 diabetic patients out of which 320 were treated with insulin and 41 were treated with diet or oral hypoglycaemic agents along with 45 non-diabetic subjects aged 11to 83 years. 57.9% of the diabetic individuals and 4.4% of the non-diabetic subjects were diagnosed with limited joint mobility. 131 of the 238 (55%) patients with non-insulin dependent diabetes and 60 of the 82 subjects (73%) receiving insulin therapy who developed diabetes after the age of 35 years had limited joint mobility LJM. Significant association ($p \leq 0.001$) of LJM and duration of diabetes was observed in insulin dependent diabetes mellitus subjects of less than 40 years of age. In diabetic patients with neuropathy under the age of 40 years and less than 20 years of diabetes LJM was significantly more frequent ($p \leq 0.03$) than those without neuropathy. In subjects under 40 years of age with retinopathy and less than 30 years of diabetes LJM was significantly more common ($p \leq 0.005$).

2.4   Handgrip Strength and Quality of Life in Patients with Type-2 Diabetes Mellitus

Poole *et al.* (2015) conducted a cross-sectional study on non-Hispanic white adults with and without type-2 diabetes to assess factors affecting quality of life. In the study, 19 adults aged 18-75 years with type-2 diabetes and 19 healthy adults without diabetes were recruited. Information about age, ethnicity, marital status, education level, employment and current health was collected using self reported questionnaire. Grip and pinch strength were measured using adapted sphygmomanometer. A strength score of each hand was established by adding mean scores for grip, two point pinch and three point pinch strength. Results exhibited that overall quality of life for adults with type-2 diabetes was decreased in comparison to adults without type-2 diabetes and people suffering from other chronic conditions. In contrary to previous studies, no significant differences were found between the hand strength and adapted hand strength between adults with type-2 diabetes and healthy adults. They attributed this finding of their study to the higher percentage of women in the healthy control group as compared to higher percentage of men in the diabetic group. As men have greater overall strength than women, this might have resulted in negligible differences in hand strength between the diabetic and healthy adults.

Cederlund *et al.* (2007) conducted a cross sectional study to examine the effect of type-2 diabetes on hand function and activities of daily living in elderly males. The study examined 51 males with impaired glucose tolerance (IGT), 69 males with type-2 diabetes and 62 age and gender matched individuals with normal glucose tolerance (NGT). Seven tests were performed on both hands for the assessment of hand function - vibration sense, using tactilometry, Semmes-

Weinstein monofilament (SWF) testing, static two-point discrimination, shape/texture identification, Purdue Pegboard Test, grip strength with Jamar dynamometer, key pinch and pinch strength with pinch gauge. Type-2 diabetic patients more frequently experienced hand disorders such as the prayer sign and Duputyren's contracture. Reduced vibrotactile sense in index and little fingers was observed in diabetic individuals in comparison to individuals with IGT and NGT. Lesser ADL complications were seen in IGT individuals than those with NGT and DM. However, no significant differences were evaluated for grip strength between two groups. The study indicated that severe neuropathy and ADL difficulties are observed in type-2 diabetic individuals with increased duration of diabetes.

2.5   Physical Fitness Evaluation in Patients with Type -2 Diabetes Mellitus

Ozdirenc *et al.* (2003) performed physical fitness evaluation in type-2 diabetes mellitus patients. The study involved 30 type-2 diabetic patients screened after OGTT (oral glucose tolerance test) and 30 age and sex matched controls. EUROFIT Physical Fitness Test Battery was used to measure body composition, cardiopulmonary, musculoskeletal and motor fitness. Jamar dynamometer was used to measure grip strength. The analysis revealed significantly higher ($p \leq 0.05$) percent body fat in the diabetic group. 6-min walk test revealed higher systolic blood pressure and heart rate where as lower values of VO_2 max and Borg scale score in diabetic individuals ($p \leq 0.05$). The subjects motor fitness evaluation assessed significantly shorter standing time for the diabetic group ($p \leq 0.05$). Vertical jump and grip strength values were significantly lower in diabetic individuals in comparison to the control subjects. Significantly reduced body flexibility on both sides was reported in the diabetic group ($p \leq 0.05$). The study emphasized the importance of physical fitness evaluation while designing exercise programs for type-2 diabetic individuals.

Grauw *et al.* (1999) carried a cross-sectional study to assess functional health status in patients with type-2 diabetes mellitus. The study involved 127 type-2 diabetic and 127 control subjects. Functional health status was measured using two instruments- the Sickness Impact Profile and the COOP/WONCA charts (The Darmouth Primary Care Cooperative Research Network and the World Organization of National Colleges, Acadamies and Academics Associations of General Practitioners/ Family physicians). The results showed significantly higher values of body mass index (p≤0.005), prevalence of cardiovascular morbidity (p≤0.002) and eye diseases (p≤0.001) in type-2 diabetic individuals. In type-2 diabetic individuals functional impairment is significantly more common in type-2 diabetic patients (p≤0.0001). Functional impairment was 2.46 times more likely to present in diabetic individuals than controls and associated with cardiovascular morbidity, locomotor morbidity, and diabetes.

2.6 Effects of Training Programmes on Handgrip Strength in Patients with Type-2 Diabetes Mellitus

Agbonlahor and Adebisi (2017) conducted a cross-sectional study to assess the effect of strength training programme on hand function in type-2 diabetic patients. Handgrip strength was measured using electronic hand dynamometer and pinch strength with mechanical pinch gauge before and after 12-week strengthening programme. The strength training programme was performed three times per week and each session lasted for 50 minutes at 70% one repetition maximum (70% 1RM) and 8 sets of repetition for each muscle group and rest of 3 minutes between sets. Upper limbs muscle strengthening was the main focus of the strength training programme to improve hand function in diabetic individuals. Noticeable difference was observed in grip strength in diabetic and non-diabetic individuals before the training session. Significant improvement of handgrip strength in diabetic individuals (p≤0.001) was observed after the strength training programme. The study revealed the importance of strength training programme in improving hand function in patients with type-2 diabetes mellitus.

Thorat and Ganvir (2015) studied the strength training effectiveness on hand function in diabetic neuropathy patients. The study involved 10 diabetes mellitus patients (males=4, females=6) aged 30-60 years with duration of diabetes of more than 25 years. Jamar hand-held dynamometer was used to assess grip strength before and after strength training program. Four weeks strength training was administered using spring hand dynamometer, rubber band and squeeze ball. The study showed statistically significant improvement of right and left handgrip strength before and after strength training program. Improved hand function in patients with diabetic neuropathy was attributed to improved muscle strength, flexibility and glycemic control with strength training program.

Herriott *et al.* (2004) evaluated the effect of flexibility and resistance training of 8-weeks in type-2 diabetic elderly individuals. The participants included 9 diabetic subjects (5 men and 4 women) with mean age of 50.6 ±2.8 years and 10 non-diabetic sedentary controls (6 men and 4 women) with mean age of 54.7 ±2.8 years. The flexibility tests involved inclinometer tests, shoulder ROM, prayer sign and modified sit and reach tests. Resistance training was performed on eight different resistance training machines on 3 non-consecutive days of the week over an 8-week period. Flexibility exercises were performed for 10-30 seconds each that stretched the major muscles groups of the chest, shoulder and legs. Both before and after training individual measures of flexibility were similar between the type-2 diabetic and control group. Modified sit and reach, left knee flexion and left hip flexion flexibility measures improved significantly in the diabetic group, where as no significant improvement was seen in control subjects. Over all lower body flexibility increased significantly more than control subjects. Significant strength gains were exhibited in both groups.

2.7   Handgrip Strength in Elderly Adults

Kalyani *et al.* (2015) observed the effect of potential sex differences on the fasting and post challenge glucose levels association with grip strength among elderly diabetic adults. The measurements of fasting plasma glucose were taken in 1019 women and 636 men and of two hour glucose (2HG) levels after 75g oral glucose tolerance test in 870 women and 559 men. The mean age of these subjects was seventy-one years. Hand held dynamometer was used to measure dominant handgrip strength on three different visits over a period of seven years. Amongst men after adjusting for age, education, height, weight, peripheral neuropathy, physical activity and other factors, each SD (SD=17mg/dl) increase in fasting plasma glucose was related with continuous decrease in grip strength, where as no relation of two hour glucose level was observed with grip strength. In women, no association was observed between fasting plasma glucose and two hour plasma glucose level with grip strength. The study revealed that in elderly males, elevated fasting plasma glucose levels were related to persistently lower grip strength but not in females.

Sasaki *et al.* (2007) conducted a study on middle aged and elderly individuals of age group between 35-70 years consisting of men (n=1695) and women (n=3217) to establish grip strength as an indicator of cause specific mortality. Measurements of handgrip strength were be extended up to a period of two years viz., from June 1970 to July 1972 and follow up for mortality was done till the end of 1999. The results of their findings depicted that the subjects with higher grip strength, had low mortality rates. Further, it has been reported that in men both low and high handgrip strength values, are indicators of incident mortality. However in case of women, low grip strength values pose a risk for premature death but the high grip strength values were not shielding.

MATERIALS AND METHODS

3.1   Design of Study

A successful research involves an efficient study design. The current research involved a cross-sectional study design.

3.1.1 Punjab and its people

The name Punjab has been given on the names of the five rivers (i.e. Sutlej, Ravi, Beas, Chenab and Jhelum) which flew through the region before Indo-Pak partition. The Indian Punjab now has Sutlej, Ravi and Beas. Punjab is the 20th largest Indian state according to the area covered by it. Punjab covers about 50,632 square kilometres of area. It is the main state of North India, bordered by Jammu and Kashmir to the North, on the East by Himachal Pradesh, with Haryana on South and South East and on South West by Rajasthan. On the basis of population, Punjab is the 16th largest state, consisting of twenty two districts. According to 2011 census, the population of Punjab is 27,704,236, with a sex ratio of 846:1000. The male population of Punjab is 14,639,465 and female population is 13,103,873. The major population of Punjab consists of Sikhs which form 57.7% of total population, followed by Hindus which constitute 38.5% share of population. The Union Territory of Punjab is Chandigarh.

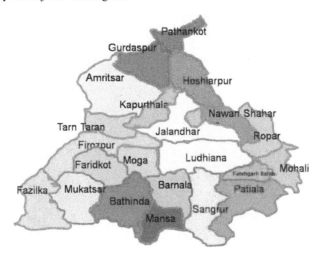

Figure 3.1: Map of Punjab state

37

3.1.2 Selection of sample

Study group consisted of 576 confirmed cases of type-2 diabetes mellitus (251 males, 325 females) with a mean duration of diabetes of more than 5 years, and 529 controls (241 males, 288 females) without any history of glucose intolerance. The subjects' ranged from age group of 30-65 years. The subjects' age was estimated from their birth date. The subjects with any history of pain and musculoskeletal problems in the shoulder, arm or hand, documented history of trauma or brachial plexus injury, or cervical radiculopathy in the previous 6 months of the commencement of the study were excluded from the study. The consent was obtained from the subjects in written format. The data were collected in morning (between 8 AM to 12 noon) under natural environmental condition. The institutional ethical committee approved the study.

3.1.3 Sample size calculation

For the calculation of sample size, the following formula was applied:

$$n = \frac{t^2 * p\,(1-p)}{m^2}$$

Where n = sample size

t = 95% CI (standard value of 1.96)

p = frequency of dependent variables in the population

m = margin of error %.

3.1.4 Inclusion criteria:

1. Only type-2 diabetes mellitus patients were considered as samples.

2. Age group 40-65 years was considered.

3. Samples were taken from Amritsar.

4. The patients suffering from diabetes mellitus for more than 5 years.

3.1.5 Exclusion Criteria:

1. Patients having any hand injury were excluded.

2. Patients below the age of 40 years and above the age of 65 years were excluded.

3. People suffering from any disease other than type-2 diabetes were excluded from the study.

3.1.6 Place of the study

Study was carried out in Civil Hospital Amritsar, Civil Hospital Ajnala, Clinic of Dr. Rohit Kapoor, Rani Ka Bagh, Camp at Attari, Amritsar.

Table 3.1

Distribution of the Subjects

Population	Absolute No.	Percent
Diabetic males	251	22.71
Diabetic females	325	29.41
Control males	241	21.80
Control females	288	26.06
Total	**1105**	**100.0**

3.2 Methods

3.2.1 Procedure of data collection

The individuals participating in the study were made aware about the study purpose an informed consent was taken from them. The assessment of all the anthropometric parameters was done on each and individuals fallowing Lohman *et al.* (1988). Handgrip strength was measured from both the left and right sides.

a. Measurement of dominant and non-dominant handgrip strength

Using a standard adjustable digital dynamometer (Takei Scientific Instruments Co., Ltd., Japan) dominant and non-dominant handgrip strength was measured. It was done at standing position with elbow in full extension. The subject was instructed to exert maximum force on the dynamometer three times and the maximum value was recorded in kg. Handheld handgrip strength dynamometer was calibrated before each measurement.

b.   **Anthropometric measurements**

The following anthropometric parameters were assessed:

1.   **Height vertex (Hv)**

Using the anthropometric rod, the height vertex of the subject was measured from floor to the vertex of the subject in cm.

2.   **Body weight (Bw)**

Using the digital weighing machine, body weight of the subject was measured in kg with minimum clothing and without shoes.

3.   **Body mass index (BMI)**

Body mass index of the subject was derived by dividing the body weight (in kg) by square of height vertex (in meters). Hence it was represented by:

BMI= Body mass (kg) / Height $(m)^2$

4.   **Upper arm circumference (Uac)**

Using steel tape, the maximum circumference of the upper arm of the subject was measured in cm.

5.   **Waist circumference (Wc)**

Using steel tape, the maximum circumference of the waist of the subject was measured in cm.

6.   **Hip circumference (Hc)**

Using steel tape, the maximum circumference of the hip of the subject was measured in cm.

7.   **Biceps skinfold (Bsf)**

Using Harpenden skinfold caliper, the skinfold on the biceps muscle of the subject was measured in mm.

8.   **Triceps skinfold (Tsf)**

Using Harpenden skinfold caliper, the skinfold over the triceps muscle of the subject was measured in mm.

9.   **Upper arm length (Ual)**

Using anthropometer rod, the upper arm length was measured from acromion to radiale of the subject in cm.

10.   **Forearm length (Fl)**

Using anthropometer rod, the forearm length was measured from radiale to stylion of the subject in cm.

11.   **Total arm length (Tal)**

Using anthropometer rod, the total arm length was measured from acromion to dactylion of the subject in cm.

12.   **Hand length (Hl)**

Using sliding caliper, the hand length of the subject was measured from the base line of the crease of the wrist to the tip of the middle finger was measured in cm.

13.   **Hand Breadth (Hb)**

Using sliding caliper, the hand breadth of the subject was measured from the widest point of the head of the first metacarpal to the fifth metacarpal in cm.

14.   **Hand span (Hs)**

Using sliding caliper, the hand span of the subject was measured in cm from the tip of the thumb to the tip of the little finger, when the palm is maximally stretched.

15.   **Arm muscle girth (Amg)**

It was derived from the formula given below after Mcardle *et al.* (2001):

Arm muscle area (cm) = $[G_{arm} - (\pi Sf_{tri})]$.

16.   **Arm muscle area Ama)**

It was derived from the formula given below after Mcardle *et al.* (2001):

Arm muscle area (cm2) = [$G_{arm} - (\pi Sf_{tri})$] / 4π.

17. **Arm area (Aa)**

It was derived from the formula given below after Mcardle *et al.* (2001):

Arm area (cm2) = $(G_{arm})^2 / 4\pi$.

18. **Arm fat area (Afa)**

It was derived from the formula given below after Mcardle *et al.* (2001):

Arm fat area (cm²) = arm area - arm muscle area

19. **Arm fat index (Afi)**

It was derived from the formula given below after Mcardle *et al.* (2001):

Arm fat index = arm fat area / arm area.

20. **Waist to hip ratio (W/Hr)**

This ratio was calculated by the following formula:

Waist to hip ratio = Waist circumference / Hip circumference.

21. **% Body fat** (Siri, 1956) (% Bf)

The %bf was calculated by the following formula:

Percent body fat = {(4.95/Body density)-4.5}*100

Body density (Durnin and Womersley, 1974)

Body density for men = 1.1610 - 0.0632 logΣ4

Body density for women = 1.1581 – 0.0720 logΣ4

22. **% Lean body mass (% Lbm)**

The % lbm was calculated by the following formula:

Percent lean body mass = 100 - percent body fat.

3.3 **Statistical Analysis**

The statistical formulae used in the present study were described below:

3.3.1 **Arithmetic mean ($\sqrt{X}$)**

The arithmetic mean was calculated by the formula given below:

$$\sqrt{X} = X / N$$

Where,

$$\sqrt{X} \quad = \quad \text{arithmetic mean}$$

$$X \quad = \quad \text{sum of all variables}$$

$$N \quad = \quad \text{total number of samples}$$

3.3.2 Standard deviation (SD)

The standard deviation was calculated by the formula given below:

$$S.D. = \sqrt{\frac{\Sigma (X - \bar{X})^2}{N}}$$

Where

$$S.D. \quad = \quad \text{Standard deviation}$$

$$X \quad = \quad \text{Individual value of the variables}$$

$$\bar{X} \quad = \quad \text{Mean of variables}$$

3.3.3 Standard error (S.E.)

It reflects level of the sampling error. SE may be calculated with the formula given below:

$$S.E. = \frac{\sqrt{S.D.}}{N}$$

Where

$$S.D. \quad = \quad \text{Standard deviation}$$

$$N \quad = \quad \text{Total number of samples}$$

3.3.4 Student's t-test

The Student's t-test was calculated by the formula given below:

$$t = \frac{\sqrt{\bar{X}_1 - \bar{X}_2}}{(S.E._1)^2 + (S.E._2)^2}$$

Where

t   =   Student's t test

$\overline{X}_1$ =   Mean of 1st group of samples

$\overline{X}_2$ =   Mean of group of samples

S.E.$_1$ =   Standard error of 1st 1st group of samples

S.E.$_2$ =   Standard error of 2nd group of samples

3.3.5 Correlation

Karl Pearson's product moment correlation coefficients (r) were calculated the following formula:

$$r = \frac{N\sum (A \times B) - \sum A \times \sum B}{\sqrt{[N\sum A^2 - (\sum A)^2][N\sum B^2 - \sum B)^2]}}$$

$\sum A$ =   Sum of variables A

$\sum B$ =   Sum of variables B

DF   =   N-2

The level of significance was $p < 0.05$.

3.3.6 Regression analysis

To quantify the correlation between the handgrip strength (dependent variable) with selected anthropometric variables (independent variables), regression analysis was applied.

Linear regression

It was calculated with the equation given below:

$$y = a + bx$$

Where, y was the value of the handgrip strength (dependent variable) and x was the value of anthropometric (independent) variables. Further:

$$b = \frac{\text{sum of } xy - \{(\text{sum } x)\,(\text{sum } y)n\}}{\text{sum } x^2\,(\text{sum } x)^2/n}$$

$$a= [(\text{sum } y)/n]-[b(\text{sum } x)/n]$$

Multiple regression

It was calculated by the regression analysis given below:

$$y = a + b_1x_1 + b_2x_2\ldots\ldots\ldots + b_n x_n$$

Where, $x_1, x_2 \ldots x_n$ were the independent variables, $b_1, b_2 \ldots$ bn were the regression coefficients of $x_1, x_2 \ldots x_n$ respectively (dependent variable).

RESULTS

4.1 Comparison of Handgrip Strength and Selected Anthropometric Variables

Table 4.1 showed the comparison of handgrip strength and selected anthropometric variables in patients with type-2 diabetes mellitus and controls. Diabetic individuals had significantly lower ($p \leq 0.001$) mean values in dominant handgrip strength (Dhgs) (t=5.10) and non-dominant handgrip strength (Ndhgs) (t=5.19), and significantly higher ($p \leq 0.03-0.001$) mean values in age (t=3.27), upper arm circumference (Uac) (t=2.81), waist circumference (Wc) (t=5.09), hip circumference (Hc) (t=2.56), biceps skinfold (Bsf) (t=2.49), triceps skinfold (Tsf) (t=2.95), arm muscle girth (Amg) (t=2.75), arm muscle area (Ama) (t=2.64), arm area (Aa) (t=2.31) and arm fat area (Afa) (t=2.17) than their control counterparts.

The comparison of handgrip strength and selected anthropometric variables of diabetic males and females aged 30-65 years was shown in table 4.2. Diabetic males had significantly greater ($p \leq 0.04-0.001$) mean values in Dghs (t=18.90), Ndhgs (t=17.54), age (t=4.49), height vertex (Hv) (t=4.74), bodyweight (Bw) (t=10.39), Wc (t=4.13), Hc (t=2.09), Ual (t=14.80), Fal (t=10.77), Tal (t=15.90), Hl (t=11.67), Hb (t=14.89), Hs (t=15.49), Afa (t=2.12), Afi (t=7.44),W-hr (t=3.82), and % Lbm (t=25.32), and significantly lower (p<0.001) mean values in BMI (t=2.09), Bsf (t=5.29), Tsf (t=5.51), Amg (t=6.37), Ama (t=6.61) and % Bf (t=25.32) than their female counterparts.

Table 4.3 showed the comparison of handgrip strength and selected anthropometric variables of diabetic and control males aged 30-65 years. Diabetic males had significantly greater ($p \leq 0.03-0.001$) mean values, in age (t=2.63), Bw (t=2.61), BMI (t=2.97), Uac (t=4.56), Hc (t=3.01), Bsf (t=2.44), Tsf (t=2.25), Aa (t=4.40), Afa (t=4.42), Afi (t=2.52), W-hr (t=3.32) and % Bf (t=2.97) and significantly lower ($p \leq 0.001$) mean values in Dhgs (t=6.09cm), Ndhgs (t=5.35) and % Lbm (t=2.97) than their control counterparts.

The comparison of handgrip strength and selected anthropometric variables of diabetic and control females aged 30-65 years was shown in table 4.4. Diabetic females had significantly greater (p≤0.01-0.001) mean values in Wc (t=2.85), Tsf (t=2.57), Amg (t=2.83) and Ama (t=2.89), and significantly lower (p≤0.001) mean values in Dhgs (t=4.27) and Ndhgs (t=5.94).

Table 4.5 showed the comparison of handgrip strength and selected anthropometric variables in urban and rural male diabetic patients. Rural male diabetic patients had significantly higher (p≤0.04-0.001) mean values in Dhgs (t=2.51), Bw (t=2.24), BMI (t=2.57), Wc (t=3.76), Hb (t=2.12), W-hr (t=4.19) and % Bf (t=2.57), and significantly lower (p≤0.01) mean value in % Lbm (t=2.57) than their urban male diabetic counterparts.

The comparison of handgrip strength and selected anthropometric variables in urban and rural female diabetic patients was presented in table 4.6. Urban female diabetic patients had significantly lower (p≤0.02) mean value only in Hb (t=2.46) than their rural female diabetic counterparts.

Table 4.7 showed the comparison of handgrip strength and selected anthropometric variables in urban male and female diabetic patients. Urban male diabetic patients had significantly higher (p≤0.03-0.001) mean values in Dhgs (t=15.54), Ndhgs (t=14.69), age (t=4.17), Hv (t=30.66), Bw (t=7.42), Wc (t=2.35), Ual (t=13.03), Fal (t=10.27), Tal (t=13.71), Hl (t=10.37), Hb (t=13.38), Hs (t=13.77), Afi (t=6.23), W-hr (t=2.21), and % Lbm (t=23.54), and significantly lower (p≤0.001) mean values in BMI (t=5.10), Bsf (t=5.66), Tsf (t=5.76), Amg (t=6.45), Ama (t=6.63) and % Bf (t=23.54) than their urban female diabetic counterparts.

The comparison of handgrip strength and selected anthropometric variables in rural male and female diabetic patients was given in table 4.8. Rural male diabetic patients had significantly higher (p≤0.04-0.001) mean values in Dhgs (t=11.20), Ndhgs (t=9.79), Hv (t=14.35), Bw (t=5.90), Uac (t=2.11), Wc (t=4.27), Hc (t=2.21), Ual (t=7.11), fore arm length (t=4.44), Tal (t=8.24), Hl (t=5.37), Hb (t=6.96), Hs (t=7.09), Aa (t=2.21), Afa (t=2.51), Afi (t=4.18), W-hr (t=4.05) and % Lbm (t=10.07), and significantly lower (p<0.001) mean value in ,%Bf (t=10.07) than their rural female counterparts.

47

4.2   One way ANOVA of Handgrip Strength and Selected Anthropometric Variables in Patients with Type-2 Diabetes Mellitus and Controls

Table 4.9 described the one way analysis of variance of handgrip strength and selected anthropometric variables in patients with type-2 diabetes mellitus and controls. Statistically significant ($p \leq 0.001$) between-group differences were found in all the variables studied, except W-hr among these four sets of population.

4.3   Correlations of Handgrip Strength with Selected Anthropometric Variables in   Male and Female Patients with Type-2 Diabetes Mellitus

Table 4.10 showed the correlation coefficients of Dhgs with selected anthropometric variables in male and female type-2 diabetic patients aged 30-65 years. In diabetic males, positively significant correlations ($p \leq 0.018$-0.001) of Dhgs were observed with Ndhgs, Bw, BMI, Wc, Tal, Hb, Hs, W-hr, and % Bf, while negatively significant correlations ($p \leq 0.018$-0.001) were noted with age and % Lbm. In diabetic females, positively significant correlations ($p \leq 0.05$-0.001) of Dhgs were observed with all the variables studied, except age, Hc, Fal and Afi, while negatively significant correlation ($p \leq 0.001$) was observed only with age. In combined male and female diabetic patients, positively significant correlations ($p < 0.028$-0.001) of Dhgs were observed with all variables studied, except age, BMI, Bsf, Tsf, Amg, Ama and % Bf, while negatively significant correlations ($p \leq 0.04$-0.0001) were observed with age, Bsf, Amg, Ama and % Bf.

The correlation coefficients of Ndhgs with selected anthropometric variables in male and female type-2 diabetic patients aged 30-65 years were shown in table 4.19. In diabetic males, positively significant correlations ($p \leq 0.035$-0.001) of Ndhgs were observed with Bw, BMI, Wc, Tal, Hb, Hs, W-hr, and % Bf, while negatively significant correlations ($p \leq 0.035$-0.001) were observed with age and % Lbm. In diabetic females, positively significant correlations ($p \leq 0.021$-0.001) of Ndhgs were observed with all variables studied, except age, Hc, Bsf, Afi and % Lbm, while negatively significant correlations ($p \leq 0.009$-0.001) were found with age and % Lbm. In combined male and female diabetic patients, positively significant correlations ($p \leq 0.01$-0.001) of Ndhgs were noted with all variables studied,   except age, BMI,

Bsf, Tsf, Amg and % Bf, while negatively significant correlations (p≤0.046-0.001) were found with age, Bsf, Tsf, Amg, Ama and % Bf.

4.4. Linear Regressions of Handgrip Strength with Selected Anthropometric Variables in Male and Female Patients with Type-2 Diabetes Mellitus

Table 4.11 showed the linear regression analysis (R^2) of Dhgs with selected anthropometric variables in patients with type-2 diabetes mellitus. In diabetic males, significant correlations (p<0.05-0.001) of Dhgs were noted with Ndhgs, age, Bw, BMI, Wc,Tal, Hl, Hb, Hs, W-hr, % Bf and % Lbm. In diabetic females, significant correlations (p<0.02-0.001) were found with all the variables studied, except Fal and Afi. In combined males and female diabetic patients, significant correlations (p<0.03-0.001) were observed with all the variables studied, except age, BMI and Tsf.

The linear regression coefficients (Beta) of Dhgs with selected anthropometric variables in patients with type-2 diabetes mellitus were given in table 4.12. In diabetic males, significant correlations (p<0.05-0.001) were found with Ndhgs, age, BMI, Tal, Hb, Hs, W-hr, % Bf and % Lbm. In diabetic females, significant correlations (p<0.05-0.001) were noted with all the variables studied, except Hc and Afi. In combined male and female diabetic patients, significant correlations (p<0.05-0.001) were observed with all the variables studied, except BMI and Bsf.

Table 4.20 showed the linear regression analysis (R^2) of Ndhgs with selected anthropometric variables in patients with type-2 diabetes mellitus. In diabetic males, significant correlations (p<0.01-0.001) of Ndhgs were found with Dhgs, age, Bw, BMI, Wc, Tal, Hb, Hs, W-hr, % Bf and % Lbm. In diabetic females, significant correlations (p<0.017-0.001) were observed with all the variables studied, except Wc, Hc and Afi. In combined male and female diabetic patients, significant correlations (p<0.013-0.001) were observed with all the variables studied, except BMI and Hc.

The linear regression coefficients (Beta) of Ndhgs with selected anthropometric variables in patients with type-2 diabetes mellitus were shown in table 4.21. In diabetic males, significant correlations (p<0.05-0.001) were noted with Dhgs, age, Bw, BMI, Wc, Tal, Hb, W-hr, % Bf and % Lbm. In diabetic females, significant correlations (p<0.05-0.001) were found with all the variables studied, except Hc, Bsf and Afi. In combined male and female diabetic patients, significant correlations (p<0.05-0.001) were found with all the variables studied, except BMI, Hc, Hs, % Bf and % Lbm.

4.5 Step-down Multiple Regression Analysis of Handgrip Strength with Selected Anthropometric Variables in Patients with Type-2 Diabetes Mellitus

Table 4.13 represented the step-down multiple regression analysis of Dhgs with selected anthropometric variables in diabetic males (R^2=0.847). Statistically significant correlations (p<0.05-0.001) were observed with Ndhgs, age, Bsf, Bsf and Hl.

The step-down multiple regression analysis of Dhgs with selected anthropometric variables in diabetic females (R^2=0.772) was shown in table 4.14. Statistically significant correlations (p<0.05-0.001) were observed with Ndhgs, age, Hv, Fal and Hl.

Table 4.15 showed the step-down multiple regression analysis of Dhgs in patients with type-2 diabetes mellitus (R^2=0.883). Statistically significant correlations (p<0.02-0.001) were found with Ndhgs, Hv, Bsf, Fal, Hl and Ama.

The step-down multiple regression analysis of Ndhgs with selected anthropometric variables in diabetic males (R^2=0.845) was shown in table 4.22. Statistically significant correlations (p<0.02-0.001) were observed with Dhgs, Bsf, Tsf, Tal and Hl.

Table 4.23 highlighted the step-down multiple regression analysis of Ndhgs with selected anthropometric variables in diabetic females (R^2=0776). Statistically significant correlations (p<0.003-0.001) were found with Dhgs, Ual, Hl and Hs.

The step-down multiple regression analysis of Ndhgs in patients with type-2 diabetes mellitus ($R^2=0.875$) was shown in Table 4.24. Statistically significant correlations ($p<0.03-0.001$) were observed with Dhgs, Wc, Tal, Hl and Amg.

4.6   Multiple   Regressions   of   Handgrip   Strength   with   Selected Anthropometric Variables in Male and Female Patients with Type-2 Diabetes Mellitus

Table 4.16 showed the multiple regression of Dhgs with selected anthropometric variables in diabetic males ($R^2=0.852$). Statistically significant correlations ($p<0.05-0.001$) of Dhgs were observed with Ndhgs, age and Bsf.

The multiple regression of Dhgs with selected anthropometric variables in diabetic females ($R^2=0.774$) was shown in table 4.17. Statistically significant correlations ($p<0.004-0.001$) of Dhgs were observed with Ndhgs and Tal.

Table 4.18 showed the multiple regression of Dhgs with selected anthropometric variables in patients with type-2 diabetes mellitus ($R^2=0.886$). Statistically significant correlations ($p<0.018-0.001$) of Dhgs were observed with Ndhgs, age, Bsf, Hl and % Lbm.

The multiple regression of Ndhgs with selected anthropometric variables in diabetic males ($R^2=0.848$) was shown in table table 4.25. Statistically significant correlations ($p<0.047-0.001$) of Ndhgs were found with Dhgs, Bsf and Hl.

Table 4.26 showed the multiple regression of Ndhgs with selected anthropometric variables in diabetic females ($R^2 = 0.769$). Statistically significant correlations ($p<0.018-0.001$) of Ndhgs were observed with Dhgs, Hl and Hs.

Themultiple regression of Ndhgs with anthropometric variables in patients with type-2 diabetes mellitus ($R^2=0.501$) was shown in table 4.27. Statistically significant correlations ($p<0.001$) of Ndhgs were observed with Dhgs, Tal and %Bf.

4.7   Correlations of Selected Anthropometric Variables in Male and Female Patients with Type-2 Diabetes Mellitus

Table 4.28 showed the correlation coefficients of age with selected anthropometric variables in male and female diabetic patients aged 30-65 years. In diabetic males, positively significant correlation ($p \leq 0.022$) of age was observed only with Ual. In diabetic females, no positively or negatively significant correlation was observed with any of the variables. In combined male and female diabetic patients, positively significant correlations ($p \leq 0.037$-0.001) of age were observed with Hv, Wc, Ual, Fal, Tal, Hs, % Bf and % Lbm.

The correlations coefficients of Hv with selected anthropometric variables in male and female diabetic patients aged 30-65 years were shown in table 4.29. In diabetic males, positively significant correlations ($p \leq 0.035$-0.001) of Hv were observed with all the variables studied, except BMI, Bsf, Afi, W-hr, % Bf and % Lbm, while negatively significant correlation ($p \leq 0.03$) was found with W-hr. In diabetic females, positively significant correlations ($p \leq 0.027$-0.001) of Hv were observed with Bw, Wc, Hc, Bsf, Tsf, Ual, Fal, Tal, Hl, Hb, Hs, Amg and Ama. In combined male and female diabetic patients, positively significant correlations ($p \leq 0.019$-0.001) of Hv were noted with all the variables studied, except BMI, Bsf, Tsf, Amg, Ama and % Bf, as they showed negatively significant correlation ($p \leq 0.031$-0.001) with Hv.

Table 4.30 showed the correlation coefficients of Bw with selected anthropometric variables in male and female diabetic patients aged 30-65 years. In diabetic males, positively significant correlations ($p \leq 0.01$) of Bw were found with all the variables studied, except Afi and % Lbm as the latter observed negatively significant correlation ($p \leq 0.001$) with Bw. In diabetic females, positively significant correlations ($p \leq 0.001$) of Bw were found with all the variables studied, except Afi, W-hr and % Lbm, while negatively significant correlation ($p \leq 0.001$) was noted with % Lbm. In combined male and female diabetic patients, positively significant correlations ($p \leq 0.017$-0.001) of Bw were observed with all the variables studied, except % Lbm which showed negatively significant correlation ($p \leq 0.001$) with Bw.

The correlation coefficients of BMI with selected anthropometric variables in male and female diabetic patients aged 30-65 years were shown in table 4.31. In diabetic males, positively significant correlations ($p \leq 0.021$-0.001) of BMI were found with all the variables studied, except Ual, Fal and Afi, while negatively significant correlation ($p \leq 0.001$) was observed with % Lbm. In diabetic males, positively significant correlations ($p \leq 0.001$) of BMI were noted with all variables studied, except Ual, Fal, Tal, Afi, W-hr, while negatively significant correlation ($p \leq 0.001$) was found with % Lbm. In combined male and female diabetic patients, positively significant correlations ($p \leq 0.002$-0.001) of BMI were noted with Uac, Bsf, Tsf, Amg, Ama, Aa, W-hr, % Bf, while negatively significant correlations ($p \leq 0.024$-0.001) were found with Tal, Afa and % Lbm.

Table 4.32 showed the correlation coefficients of Uac with selected anthropometric variables in male and female diabetic patients aged 30-65 years. In diabetic males, positively significant correlations ($p \leq 0.006$-0.001) of Uac were observed with all the variables studied, except Ual, Fal, Tal, Afa and W-hr. In diabetic females, positively significant correlations ($p \leq 0.013$-0.001) of Uac were found with all the variables studied, except Fal, Tal, Hl and W-hr. In combined male and female diabetic patients, positively significant correlations ($p \leq 0.017$-0.001) were observed with all the variables studied, except Tal and W-hr. In all the above three groups Uac was noted negatively significant correlation ($p \leq 0.001$) with % Lbm.

The correlation coefficients of Wc with selected anthropometric variables in male and female diabetic patients aged 30-65 years were given in table 4.33. In diabetic males, positively significant correlations ($p \leq 0.001$) of Wc were noted with all the variables studied, except Ual, Fal, Tal, Hb and Afi. In diabetic females, positively significant correlations ($p \leq 0.027$-0.001) of Wc were found with all the variables studied, except Fal, Tal and Afi. In combined male and female diabetic patients, positively significant correlations of Wc ($p \leq 0.006$-0.001) were noted with all the variables studied, except % Lbm. In all the above three groups, negatively significant correlation ($p \leq 0.001$) of Wc was found with % Lbm.

Table 4.34 showed the correlation coefficients of Hc with selected anthropometric variables in male and female diabetic patients aged 30-65 years. In diabetic males, positively significant correlations (p≤0.045-0.001) of Hc were found with all the variables studied, except Tal, Hs, Afi, W-hr and % Lbm. In diabetic females, positively significant correlations (p≤0.001) of Hc were noted with all the variables studied, except Fal, Tal, Afi, W-hr and % Lbm. In combined male and female diabetic patients, positively significant correlations (p≤0.05-0.001) of Hc were observed with all the variables studied, except W-hr and % Lbm. In all the above three groups, negatively significant correlation (p≤0.001) of Hc was found with % Lbm.

The correlation coefficients of Bsf with selected anthropometric variables in male and female diabetic patient's age 30-65 years were shown in table 4.35. In diabetic males, positively significant correlations (p≤0.001) of Bsf were found with Tsf, Amg, Ama, Aa, Afa, Afi and % Bf, while negatively significant correlations (p≤0.012-0.001) were noted with Tal and % Lbm. In diabetic females, positively significant correlations (p≤0.027-0.001) of Bsf were found with all the variables studied, except Fal, Tal, Hs and W-hr, while negatively significant correlations were observed with Afi and % Lbm. In combined male and female diabetic patients, positively significant correlations (p≤0.001) of Bsf were reported with Tsf, Amg, Ama, Aa, Afa and % Bf, while negatively significant correlations (p≤0.001) were observed with Tal, Afi and % Lbm.

Table 4.36 showed the correlation coefficients of Tsf with selected anthropometric variables in male and female diabetic patients aged 30-65 years. In diabetic males, positively significant correlations (p≤0.042-0.001) of Bsf were noted with Hl, Amg, Ama, Aa, Afa, Afi and % Bf, while negatively significant correlations (p≤0.001) were found with Afi and % Lbm. In diabetic females, positively significant correlations (p≤0.004-0.001) of Bsf were observed with all of the variables studied, except Tal and W-hr, while negatively significant correlations (p≤0.001) were found with Afi and % Lbm. In combined male and female diabetic patients, positively significant correlations (p≤0.001) were reported with Amg, Ama, Aa, Afa and % Bf, while negatively significant correlations (p≤0.009-0.001) were observed with Tal, Afi and % Lbm.

The correlation coefficients of Ual with selected anthropometric variables in male and female diabetic patients aged 30-65 years were shown in table 4.37. In diabetic males, positively significant correlations (p≤0.001) of Ual were reported with Fal, Tal, Hl, Hb and Hs. In diabetic females, positively significant correlations (p≤0.016-0.001) of Ual were noted with all the variables studied, except Afi, W-hr, % Bf and % Lbm. In combined male and female diabetic patients, positively significant correlations (p≤0.005-0.001) were reported with all the variables studied, except Amg and Ama while negatively significant correlation (p≤0.001) was observed with % Bf.

Table 4.38 showed the correlation coefficients of Fal with selected anthropometric variables in male and female diabetic patients aged 30-65 years. In diabetic males, positively significant correlations (p≤0.001) of Fal were reported with Tal, Hl and Hs, while negatively significant correlation (p≤0.001) was observed with Hb. In diabetic females, positively significant correlations (p≤0.002-0.001) were reported with Tal, Hl, Hb, Hs, Amg and Ama. In combined male and female diabetic patients, positively significant correlations (p≤0.001) of Fal were observed with Tal, Hl, Hb and Hs.

The correlation coefficients of Tal with selected anthropometric variables in male and female diabetic patients aged 30-65 years were given in table 4.39. In diabetic males and diabetic females, positively significant correlations (p≤0.001) of Tal were reported with Hl, Hb and Hs. In combined male and female diabetic patients, positively significant correlations (p≤0.002-0.001) of Tal were noted with Hl, Hb, Hs, Aa, Afi, W-hr and % Lbm, while negatively significant correlations (p≤0.002-0.001) were observed with Amg and % Bf.

Table 4.40 showed the correlation coefficients of Hl with selected anthropometric variables in male and female diabetic patients aged 30-65 years. In diabetic males, positively significant correlations (p<0.021-0.001) of Hl were reported with Hb, Hs, Ama, Aa, Afa and % Bf, while negatively significant correlation (p≤0.021) was found with % Lbm. In diabetic females, positively significant correlations (p≤0.001) of Hl were found with Hb, Hs, Amg, Ama and % Bf, while negatively significant correlations (p≤0.024-0.001) were observed with

55

Afi and % Lbm. In combined male and female diabetic patients, positively significant correlations (p≤0.001) of Hl were reported with Hb, Hs, Aa, Afa and % Lbm, while negatively significant correlation was noted with % Bf.

The correlation coefficients of Hb with selected anthropometric variables in male and female diabetic patients aged 30-65 years were given in table 4.41. In diabetic males, positively significant correlations (p≤0.017-0.001) of Hb were reported with Hs, Aa, Afa, W-hr, and % Bf, while negatively significant correlation (p≤0.001) was found with % Lbm. In diabetic females, positively significant correlations (p≤0.001) were observed with Hs, Amg, Ama, Aa, Afa and % Bf, while negatively significant correlation (p≤0.001) was found with % Lbm. In combined male and female diabetic patients, positively significant correlations (p≤0.001) of Hb were noted with Hs, Aa, Afa, Afi, W-hr and % Lbm, while negatively significant correlation (p≤0.001) was observed only with % Bf.

Table 4.42 showed the correlation coefficients of Hs with selected anthropometric variables in male and female diabetic patients aged 30-65 years. In diabetic males, positively significant correlations (p≤0.009-0.001) of Hs were found with Aa, Afa and % Bf. In diabetic females, positively significant correlations (p≤0.019-0.001) of Hs were reported with Amg, Ama, Aa, Afa, and % Bf, while negatively significant correlation (p<0.001) was found with % Lbm both in diabetic males and females. In combined male and female diabetic patients, positively significant correlations (p<0.001) of Hs were observed with Aa, Afa, Afi and % Lbm, while negatively significant correlation was found with % Bf.

The correlation coefficients of Amg with selected anthropometric variables in male and female diabetic patients aged 30-65 years were given in table 4.43. In diabetic males, females and combined male and female diabetic patients, positively significant correlations (p≤0.001) of Amg were reported with Ama, Aa, Afa and % Bf. While negatively significant correlations (p≤0.001) of Amg were observed with Afi and % Lbm in diabetic males, females and combined male and female diabetic patients.

Table 4.44 showed the correlation coefficients of Ama with selected anthropometric variables in male and female diabetic patients aged 30-65 years. In diabetic males, females and combined male and female diabetic patients, positively significant correlations (p≤0.001) of Ama were reported with Aa, Afa, and % Bf, while negatively significant correlations (p≤0.001) were observed with Afi and % Lbm in all the above three groups.

The correlation coefficients of Aa with selected anthropometric variables in male and female diabetic patients aged 30-65 years were shown in table 4.45. In diabetic males and females, positively significant correlations (p≤0.001) of Afa were found with Afa, Afi and % Bf, while negatively significant correlation (p≤0.001) was noted with % Lbm. In combined male and female diabetic patients, positively significant correlations (p≤0.001) of Aa were observed with Afa and % Bf, while negatively significant correlations (p≤0.001) were reported with Afi and % Lbm.

Table 4.46 showed the correlation coefficients of Afa with selected anthropometric variables in male and female diabetic patients aged 30-65 years. In diabetic males, diabetic females and combined male and female diabetic patients, positively significant correlations (p≤0.001) of Afa were noted with Afi and % Bf, while negatively significant correlation (p≤0.001) was observed with % Lbm.

The correlation coefficients of Afi with selected anthropometric variables in male and female diabetic patients aged 30-65 years were shown in table 4.47. In diabetic males and diabetic females, no positive or negatively significant correlation of Afi was reported with any of the variables. In combined male and female diabetic patients, positively significant correlation (p≤0.001) of Afi was noted with % Lbm, while negatively significant correlation (p≤0.001) was observed with % Bf.

Table 4.48 showed the correlation coefficients of W-hr with selected anthropometric variables in male and female diabetic patients aged 30-65 years. In diabetic males, positively significant correlation (p≤0.001) of W-hr was found with % Bf, while negatively significant correlation (p≤0.001) was observed with % Lbm. In diabetic females and combined male and female diabetic patients, no positive or negatively significant correlations were reported with any of the variables.

The correlation coefficients of % Bf with % Lbm in male and female diabetic patients aged 30-65 years were shown in table 4.49. In diabetic males, diabetic females and combined male and female diabetic patients, negatively significant correlation (p≤0.001) of % Bf was noted with % Lbm.

Table 4.1: Comparison of handgrip strength and selected anthropometric variables in patients with type-2 diabetes mellitus and controls

Variables	Diabetic patients (n=576)		Controls (n=529)		t-value	p-value
	Mean	SD	Mean	SD		
Dhgs (kg)	18.91	5.59	21.42	9.65	5.10	<0.001
Ndhgs (kg)	16.29	5.49	18.24	6.24	5.19	<0.001
Age (years)	54.06	8.25	52.26	8.88	3.27	<0.001
Hv (cm)	162.69	8.91	161.82	8.82	1.54	0.13
Bw (kg)	71.61	11.93	70.11	12.85	1.90	0.06
BMI (kg/m²)	27.06	4.03	26.82	4.84	0.85	0.39
Uac (cm)	30.50	3.71	29.75	4.64	2.81	<0.01
Wc (cm)	99.28	10.44	95.72	11.42	5.09	<0.001
Hc (cm)	107.42	9.50	105.74	11.06	2.56	<0.01
Bsf (mm)	25.58	7.11	24.39	7.71	2.49	<0.01
Tsf (mm)	35.22	7.41	33.73	8.39	2.95	<0.001
Ual (cm)	30.68	1.92	30.46	1.96	1.76	0.08
Fal (cm)	28.40	1.99	28.24	1.87	1.29	0.20
Tal (cm)	74.85	3.97	74.68	5.03	0.61	0.54
Hl (cm)	18.48	1.20	18.41	1.05	0.91	0.36
Hb (cm)	8.51	0.62	8.51	0.64	0.15	0.88
Hs (cm)	19.74	1.61	19.67	1.79	0.72	0.48
Amg(cm)	80.10	21.17	76.17	23.63	2.75	<0.01
Ama (cm²)	56.32	16.23	53.42	18.08	2.64	<0.02
Aa (cm²)	741.02	180.69	711.70	216.21	2.31	<0.02
Afa(cm²)	684.71	173.62	658.28	207.76	2.17	<0.03
Afi	0.92	0.02	0.92	0.03	0.82	0.41
W-hr	0.92	0.06	0.92	0.40	0.12	0.91
% Bf	29.73	7.96	29.90	9.07	0.32	0.75
% Lbm	70.27	7.96	70.10	9.07	0.32	0.75

Dhgs = Dominant handgrip strength, Ndhgs = Non-dominant handgrip strength, Hv = Height vertex, Bw = Body weight, BMI = Body mass index, Uac = Upper arm circumference, Wc = Waist circumference, Hc = Hip circumference, Bsf = Biceps skinfold, Tsf = Triceps skinfold, Ual = Upper arm length, Fal = Forearm length, Tal = Total arm length, Hl = Hand length, Hb = Hand breadth, Hs = Hand span, Amg = Arm muscle girth, Ama = Arm muscle area, Aa = Arm area, Afa = Arm fat area, Afi = Arm fat index, W-hr = Waist to hip ratio, % Bf = % Body fat and % Lbm = % Lean body mass.

Table 4.2: Comparison of handgrip strength and selected anthropometric variables in diabetic males and females

Variables	Diabetic males (n=251)		Diabetic females (n=325)		t-value	p-value
	Mean	SD	Mean	SD		
Dhgs (kg)	23.23	5.16	16.04	3.69	18.90	<0.001
Ndhgs(kg)	20.35	5.32	13.60	3.63	17.54	<0.001
Age (years)	55.98	7.87	52.78	8.27	4.49	<0.001
Hv (cm)	171.68	5.53	156.72	4.74	33.63	<0.001
Bw(kg)	77.09	12.02	67.98	10.39	9.38	<0.001
BMI (kg/m²)	26.13	3.74	27.67	4.10	4.45	<0.001
Uac(cm)	30.78	3.83	30.32	3.61	1.41	0.16
Wc(cm)	101.52	10.32	97.79	10.26	4.13	<0.001
Hc(cm)	108.46	9.18	106.73	9.66	2.09	<0.04
Bsf(mm)	23.64	6.92	26.86	6.95	5.29	<0.001
Tsf(mm)	33.13	7.41	36.62	7.08	5.51	<0.001
Ual(cm)	31.94	1.63	29.84	1.61	14.80	<0.001
Fal (cm)	29.43	1.65	27.72	1.91	10.77	<0.001
Tal(cm)	77.60	3.81	73.03	2.88	15.90	<0.001
Hl(cm)	19.14	0.87	18.04	1.19	11.67	<0.001
Hb(cm)	8.92	0.56	8.24	0.50	14.89	<0.001
Hs(cm)	20.84	1.44	19.01	1.27	15.49	<0.001
Amg(cm)	73.24	21.02	84.66	20.04	6.37	<0.001
Ama(cm²)	50.87	16.08	59.93	15.33	6.61	<0.001
Aa (cm²)	754.95	190.38	731.77	173.63	1.46	0.14
Afa(cm²)	704.08	182.84	671.84	166.25	2.12	<0.03
Afi	0.93	0.02	0.92	0.02	7.44	<0.001
W-hr	0.94	0.06	0.92	0.06	3.82	<0.001
% Bf	22.54	5.02	34.50	5.61	25.32	<0.001
% Lbm	77.46	5.02	66.50	5.61	25.32	<0.001

Table 4.3: Comparison of handgrip strength and selected anthropometric variables in diabetic males and control males

Variables	Diabetic males (n=251)		Control males (n=241)		t-value	p-value
	Mean	SD	Mean	SD		
Dhgs (kg)	23.23	5.16	26.82	6.09	6.09	**<0.001**
Ndhgs(kg)	20.35	5.32	23.61	6.34	5.35	**<0.001**
Age (years)	55.98	7.87	53.69	8.69	2.63	**<0.01**
Hv (cm)	171.68	5.53	171.88	4.70	0.37	0.71
Bw (kg)	77.09	12.02	73.82	11.51	2.61	**<0.01**
BMI (kg/m²)	26.13	3.74	24.96	3.63	2.97	**<0.001**
Uac (cm)	30.78	3.83	28.91	3.97	4.53	**<0.001**
Wc (cm)	101.52	10.32	96.75	9.23	4.56	**<0.001**
Hc (cm)	108.46	9.18	105.67	8.16	3.01	**<0.001**
Bsf (mm)	23.64	6.92	21.92	6.33	2.44	**<0.02**
Tsf (mm)	33.13	7.41	31.36	7.44	2.25	**<0.03**
Ual (cm)	31.94	1.63	31.99	1.67	0.30	0.76
Fal (cm)	29.43	1.65	29.58	1.51	0.88	0.38
Tal (cm)	77.60	3.81	77.86	3.58	0.65	0.51
Hl (cm)	19.14	0.87	19.22	0.76	0.95	0.34
Hb (cm)	8.92	0.56	8.99	0.54	1.16	0.25
Hs (cm)	20.84	1.44	20.74	1.85	0.57	0.57
Amg(cm)	73.24	21.02	69.55	21.93	1.63	0.11
Ama (cm²)	50.87	16.08	48.46	17.08	1.38	0.17
Aa (cm²)	754.95	190.38	668.46	178.58	4.40	**<0.001**
Afa(cm²)	704.08	182.84	620.00	175.04	4.42	**<0.001**
Afi	0.93	0.02	0.92	0.04	2.52	**<0.01**
W-hr	0.94	0.06	0.92	0.05	3.32	**<0.001**
% Bf	22.54	5.02	20.98	4.87	2.97	**<0.001**
% Lbm	77.46	5.02	79.02	4.87	2.97	**<0.001**

Table 4.4: Comparison of handgrip strength and selected anthropometric variables in diabetic females and control females

Variables	Diabetic females (n=325)		Control females (n=288)		t-value	p-value
	Mean	SD	Mean	SD		
Dhgs (kg)	16.04	3.69	18.57	9.96	4.27	**<0.001**
Ndhgs(kg)	13.60	3.63	15.40	3.89	5.94	**<0.001**
Age (years)	52.78	8.27	51.51	8.90	1.83	0.07
Hv (cm)	156.72	4.74	156.51	5.05	0.54	0.59
Bw (kg)	67.98	10.39	68.15	13.10	0.18	0.86
BMI (kg/m²)	27.67	4.10	27.79	5.11	0.32	0.75
Uac (cm)	30.32	3.61	30.20	4.90	0.36	0.72
Wc (cm)	97.79	10.26	95.18	12.40	2.85	**<0.01**
Hc (cm)	106.73	9.66	105.77	12.33	1.07	0.29
Bsf (mm)	26.86	6.95	25.70	8.05	1.92	0.06
Tsf (mm)	36.62	7.08	34.99	8.60	2.57	<0.01
Ual (cm)	29.84	1.61	29.65	1.59	1.47	0.14
Fal (cm)	27.72	1.91	27.54	1.64	1.26	0.21
Tal (cm)	73.03	2.88	73.00	4.87	0.09	0.93
Hl (cm)	18.04	1.19	17.99	0.92	0.64	0.52
Hb (cm)	8.24	0.50	8.25	0.54	0.26	0.79
Hs (cm)	19.01	1.27	19.10	1.46	0.75	0.45
Amg(cm)	84.66	20.04	79.66	23.79	2.83	**<0.01**
Ama (cm²)	59.93	15.32	56.04	18.06	2.89	**<0.001**
Aa (cm²)	731.77	173.63	734.52	230.68	0.17	0.87
Afa(cm²)	671.84	166.25	678.48	220.73	0.42	0.67
Afi	0.92	0.02	0.92	0.03	1.46	0.14
W-hr	0.92	0.06	0.93	0.50	0.34	0.73
% Bf	34.50	5.61	34.60	7.01	0.20	0.84
% Lbm	65.50	5.61	65.40	7.01	0.20	0.84

Table 4.5: Comparison of handgrip strength and selected anthropometric variables in urban and rural male diabetic patients

Variables	Urban male diabetic patients (n=165)		Rural male diabetic patients (n=86)		t-value	p-value
	Mean	SD	Mean	SD		
Dhgs (kg)	22.75	5.08	24.80	5.18	2.51	<0.01
Ndhgs (kg)	20.02	5.31	21.41	5.28	1.64	0.10
Age (years)	55.90	7.58	56.22	8.81	0.25	0.81
Hv (cm)	171.77	5.22	171.37	6.46	0.45	0.65
Bw (kg)	76.08	10.92	80.35	14.71	2.24	<0.03
BMI (kg/m²)	25.77	3.45	27.29	4.40	2.57	<0.01
Uac (cm)	30.55	3.68	31.49	4.24	1.54	0.13
Wc (cm)	100.10	9.41	106.13	11.78	3.76	<0.001
Hc (cm)	108.07	8.88	109.74	10.10	1.13	0.26
Bsf (mm)	23.42	6.45	24.36	8.28	0.85	0.40
Tsf (mm)	32.84	6.92	34.06	8.82	1.03	0.31
Ual (cm)	31.86	1.62	31.19	1.66	1.26	0.21
Fal (cm)	29.34	1.65	29.72	1.65	1.42	0.16
Tal (cm)	77.32	3.64	78.53	4.21	2.01	<0.05
Hl (cm)	19.13	0.84	19.18	0.98	0.33	0.75
Hb (cm)	8.88	0.55	9.07	0.58	2.12	<0.04
Hs (cm)	20.83	1.42	20.86	1.51	0.13	0.90
Amg(cm)	72.56	19.88	75.43	24.43	0.85	0.39
Ama (cm²)	50.39	15.28	52.44	18.53	0.80	0.43
Aa (cm²)	743.35	181.51	792.48	214.26	1.62	0.11
Afa(cm²)	692.96	175.88	740.05	201.38	1.61	0.11
Afi	0.93	0.02	0.93	0.02	0.92	0.36
W-hr	0.93	0.06	0.97	0.07	4.19	<0.001
% Bf	22.06	4.62	24.10	5.90	2.57	<0.01
% Lbm	77.94	4.62	75.90	5.90	2.57	<0.01

Table 4.6: Comparison of handgrip strength and selected anthropometric variables in urban and rural female diabetic patients

Variables	Urban female diabetic patients (n=229)		Rural female diabetic patients (n=96)		t-value	p-value
	Mean	SD	Mean	SD		
Dhgs (kg)	16.02	3.70	16.11	3.67	0.19	0.85
Ndhgs (kg)	13.51	3.67	13.86	3.52	0.75	0.46
Age (years)	52.58	8.16	53.41	8.63	0.77	0.44
Hv (cm)	156.59	4.71	157.13	4.84	0.88	0.38
Bw (kg)	68.09	10.55	67.61	9.91	0.36	0.72
BMI (kg/m²)	27.37	3.84	27.77	4.18	0.75	0.46
Uac (cm)	30.40	3.68	30.07	3.39	0.69	0.49
Wc (cm)	97.73	10.43	97.98	9.80	0.19	0.85
Hc (cm)	106.98	9.79	105.92	9.28	0.85	0.40
Bsf (mm)	27.25	6.90	25.65	7.01	1.78	0.08
Tsf (mm)	36.90	7.06	35.72	7.10	1.29	0.20
Ual (cm)	29.78	1.56	30.00	1.75	1.05	0.30
Fal (cm)	27.68	1.59	27.86	2.68	0.74	0.46
Tal (cm)	72.90	2.87	73.41	2.88	1.38	0.17
Hl (cm)	18.00	1.22	18.17	1.08	1.10	0.27
Hb (cm)	8.20	0.47	8.36	0.56	2.46	**0.02**
Hs (cm)	18.97	1.29	19.14	1.24	1.03	0.31
Amg (cm)	85.48	19.95	82.10	20.24	1.31	0.19
Ama (cm²)	60.56	15.24	57.98	15.50	1.31	0.19
Aa (cm²)	735.91	176.91	718.89	164.45	0.76	0.45
Afa (cm2)	675.34	169.33	660.91	156.81	0.67	0.50
Afi	0.92	0.02	0.92	0.02	0.77	0.44
W-hr	0.91	0.06	0.92	0.05	1.52	0.13
% Bf	34.64	5.72	34.08	5.26	0.76	0.45
% Lbm	65.36	5.72	65.92	5.26	0.76	0.45

Table 4.7: Comparison of handgrip strength and selected anthropometric variables in urban male and female diabetic patients

Variables	Urban male diabeticpatients (n=165)		Urban female diabetic patients (n=229)		t-value	p-value
	Mean	SD	Mean	SD		
Dhgs (kg)	22.75	5.08	16.02	3.70	15.54	<0.001
Ndhgs (kg)	20.02	5.31	13.51	3.67	14.69	<0.001
Age (years)	55.90	7.58	52.58	8.16	4.17	<0.001
Hv (cm)	171.77	5.22	156.59	4.71	30.66	<0.001
Bw (kg)	76.08	10.92	68.09	10.55	7.42	<0.001
BMI (kg/m²)	25.77	3.45	27.77	4.18	5.10	<0.001
Uac (cm)	30.55	3.68	30.40	3.68	0.42	0.67
Wc (cm)	100.10	9.41	97.73	10.43	2.35	<0.02
Hc (cm)	108.07	8.88	106.98	9.79	1.15	0.25
Bsf (mm)	23.42	6.45	27.25	6.90	5.66	<0.001
Tsf (mm)	32.84	6.92	36.90	7.06	5.76	<0.001
Ual (cm)	31.86	1.62	29.78	1.56	13.03	<0.001
Fal (cm)	29.34	1.65	27.68	1.59	10.27	<0.001
Tal (cm)	77.32	3.64	72.90	2.87	13.71	<0.001
Hl (cm)	19.13	0.84	18.00	1.22	10.37	<0.001
Hb (cm)	8.88	0.55	8.20	0.47	13.38	<0.001
Hs (cm)	20.83	1.42	18.97	1.29	13.77	<0.001
Amg (cm)	72.56	19.88	85.48	19.95	6.45	<0.001
Ama (cm²)	50.39	15.28	60.56	15.24	6.63	<0.001
Aa (cm²)	743.35	181.51	735.91	176.61	0.41	0.68
Afa(cm²)	692.96	175.88	735.34	169.33	1.02	0.31
Afi	0.93	0.02	0.92	0.02	6.23	<0.001
W-hr	0.93	0.06	0.91	0.06	2.21	<0.03
% Bf	22.06	4.62	34.64	5.72	23.54	<0.001
% Lbm	77.94	4.62	65.36	5.72	23.54	<0.001

Table 4.8: Comparison of handgrip strength and selected anthropometric variables in rural male and female diabetic patients

Variables	Rural male diabetic patients (n=86)		Rural female diabetic patients (n=96)		t-value	p-value
	Mean	SD	Mean	SD		
Dhgs (kg)	24.80	5.18	16.11	3.67	11.20	**<0.001**
Ndhgs (kg)	21.41	5.28	13.86	3.52	9.79	**<0.001**
Age (years)	56.22	8.81	53.41	8.63	1.80	<0.08
Hv (cm)	171.37	6.46	157.13	4.84	14.35	**<0.001**
Bw (kg)	80.35	14.71	67.61	9.91	5.90	**<0.001**
BMI (kg/m²)	27.29	4.40	27.37	3.84	0.11	0.91
Uac (cm)	31.49	4.24	30.07	3.39	2.11	**<0.04**
Wc (cm)	106.13	11.78	97.98	9.80	4.27	**<0.001**
Hc (cm)	109.74	10.10	105.92	9.28	2.21	**<0.03**
Bsf (mm)	24.36	8.28	25.65	7.01	0.96	0.34
Tsf (mm)	34.06	8.82	35.72	7.10	1.19	0.24
Ual (cm)	32.19	1.66	30.00	1.75	7.11	<0.001
Fal (cm)	29.72	1.65	27.86	2.68	4.44	<0.001
Tal (cm)	78.53	4.21	73.41	2.88	8.24	<0.001
Hl (cm)	19.18	0.98	18.17	1.08	5.37	<0.001
Hb (cm)	9.07	0.58	8.36	0.56	6.96	<0.001
Hs (cm)	20.86	1.51	19.14	1.24	7.09	<0.001
Amg (cm)	75.43	24.43	82.10	20.24	1.69	0.09
Ama (cm²)	52.44	18.53	57.98	15.50	1.84	0.07
Aa (cm²)	792.48	214.26	718.89	164.45	2.21	**<0.03**
Afa (cm²)	740.05	201.38	660.91	156.81	2.51	**<0.01**
Afi	0.93	0.02	0.92	0.02	4.18	**<0.001**
W-hr	0.97	0.07	0.92	0.05	4.05	**<0.001**
% Bf	24.10	5.90	34.08	5.26	10.07	**<0.001**
% Lbm	75.90	5.90	65.92	5.26	10.07	**<0.001**

Table 4.9: One way analysis of variance of handgrip strength and selected anthropometric variables in patients with type-2 diabetes mellitus and controls

Variables	Diabetic Males (n=251)		Diabetic Females (n=325)		Control Males (n=241)		Control Females (n=288)		F- value	p- value
	Mean	SD	Mean	SD	Mean	SD	Mean	SD		
Dhgs(kg)	23.23	5.16	16.04	3.69	26.82	6.09	18.57	9.96	110.56	≤0.001
Ndhgs (kg)	20.35	5.32	13.60	3.63	23.61	6.34	15.40	3.89	212.14	≤0.001
Age (years)	55.98	7.87	52.78	8.27	53.69	8.69	51.51	8.90	12.08	≤0.001
Ht (cm)	171.68	5.53	156.72	4.74	171.88	4.70	156.51	5.05	701.31	≤0.001
Wt (kg)	77.09	12.02	67.98	10.39	73.82	11.51	68.15	13.10	34.97	≤0.001
BMI(kg/m²)	26.13	3.74	27.67	4.10	24.96	3.63	27.79	5.11	20.31	≤0.001
Uac (cm)	30.78	3.83	30.32	3.61	28.91	3.97	30.20	4.90	6.38	≤0.001
Wc (cm)	101.52	10.32	97.79	10.26	96.75	9.23	95.18	12.40	14.63	≤0.001
Hc (cm)	108.46	9.18	106.73	9.66	105.67	8.16	105.77	12.33	3.44	≤0.001
Bs (mm)	23.64	6.92	26.86	6.95	21.92	6.33	25.70	8.05	20.00	≤0.001
Ts (mm)	33.13	7.41	36.62	7.08	31.36	7.44	34.99	8.60	19.36	≤0.001
Ual (cm)	31.94	1.63	29.84	1.61	31.99	1.67	29.65	1.59	144.12	≤0.001
Fal (cm)	29.43	1.65	27.72	1.91	29.58	1.51	27.54	1.64	90.57	≤0.001
Tal (cm)	77.60	3.81	73.03	2.88	77.86	3.58	73.00	4.87	113.85	≤0.001
Hl (cm)	19.14	0.87	18.04	1.19	19.22	0.76	17.99	0.92	106.21	≤0.001
Hb (cm)	8.92	0.56	8.24	0.50	8.99	0.54	8.25	0.54	136.44	≤0.001
Hs (cm)	20.84	1.44	19.01	1.27	20.74	1.85	19.10	1.46	108.92	≤0.001
Amg (cm)	73.24	21.02	84.66	20.04	69.55	21.93	79.66	23.79	21.82	≤0.001
Ama (cm²)	50.87	16.08	59.93	15.33	48.46	17.08	56.04	18.06	22.26	≤0.001
Aa (cm²)	754.95	190.38	731.77	173.63	668.46	178.58	734.52	230.68	6.16	≤0.001
Afa (cm²)	704.08	182.84	671.84	166.25	620.00	175.04	678.48	220.73	6.04	≤0.001
Afi	0.93	0.02	0.92	0.02	0.92	0.04	0.92	0.03	13.28	≤0.001
W-hr	0.94	0.06	0.92	0.06	0.92	0.05	0.93	0.50	0.28	0.83
%Bf	22.54	5.02	34.50	5.61	20.98	4.87	34.60	7.01	362.47	≤0.001
%Lbm	77.46	5.02	66.50	5.61	79.02	4.87	65.40	7.01	362.47	≤0.001

Table 4.10: Correlations of Dhgs with selected anthropometric variables in patients with type-2 diabetes mellitus

Variables	Diabetic males (n=251)		Diabetic females (n=325)		Combined (n=576)	
	r	p	r	p	r	p
Ndhgs (kg)	0.911	<0.001	0.866	<0.001	0.932	<0.001
Age (years)	-0.246	<0.001	-0.304	<0.001	-0.087	<0.043
Hv (cm)	0.015	0.124	0.224	<0.001	0.591	<0.001
Bw (kg)	0.187	<0.006	0.259	<0.001	0.395	<0.001
BMI (kg/m²)	0.161	<0.018	0.182	<0.001	0.009	0.829
Uac (cm)	0.089	0.193	0.162	<0.003	0.134	<0.002
Wc (cm)	0.210	<0.002	0.130	<0.019	0.238	<0.001
Hc (cm)	0.014	0.843	0.082	0.141	0.094	<0.028
Bsf (mm)	-0.045	0.513	0.144	<0.009	-0.101	<0.019
Tsf (mm)	0.014	0.836	0.211	<0.001	-0.061	0.157
Ual (cm)	0.133	0.097	0.181	<0.001	0.435	<0.001
Fal (cm)	-0.027	0.697	0.100	0.071	0.295	<0.001
Tal (cm)	0.287	<0.001	0.162	<0.003	0.505	<0.001
Hl (cm)	0.130	0.057	0.238	<0.001	0.412	<0.001
Hb (cm)	0.286	<0.001	0.188	<0.001	0.495	<0.001
Hs (cm)	0.218	<0.011	0.206	<0.001	0.486	<0.001
Amg (cm)	0.001	0.994	0.204	<0.001	-0.091	<0.035
Ama (cm²)	-0.001	0.945	0.202	<0.001	-0.099	<0.021
Aa (cm²)	0.08	0.242	0.156	<0.005	0.130	<0.002
Afa(cm²)	0.084	0.221	0.144	<0.009	0.145	<0.001
Afi	0.084	0.219	-0.057	0.302	0.201	<0.001
W-hr	0.297	<0.001	0.109	<0.05	0.258	<0.001
% Bf	0.161	<0.018	0.182	<0.001	-0.377	<0.001
% Lbm	-0.161	<0.018	-0.182	<0.001	0.377	<0.001

Table 4.11: Linear regression of Dhgs with anthropometric variables in patients with type-2 diabetes mellitus

Variables	Diabetic males (n=251)		Diabetic females (n=325)		Combined (n=576)	
	R^2	p	R^2	p	R^2	p
Ndhgs (kg)	0.83	<0.001	0.75	<0.001	0.869	<0.001
Age (years)	0.060	<0.002	0.092	<0.001	0.007	0.042
Hv (cm)	0.011	0.123	0.041	<0.001	0.348	<0.001
Bw (kg)	0.035	<0.001	0.062	<0.001	0.156	<0.001
BMI (kg/m²)	0.026	<0.01	0.033	<0.001	0.001	0.829
Uac (cm)	0.007	0.193	0.026	<0.001	0.018	<0.001
Wc (cm)	0.044	<0.001	0.016	<0.02	0.056	<0.001
Hc (cm)	0.001	0.843	0.006	<0.001	0.008	<0.02
Bsf (mm)	0.002	0.513	0.024	<0.001	0.010	<0.019
Tsf (mm)	0.002	0.835	0.044	<0.001	0.003	0.157
Ual (cm)	0.012	0.09	0.032	<0.001	0.189	<0.001
Fal (cm)	0.007	0.697	0.010	0.070	0.087	<0.001
Tal (cm)	0.088	<0.001	0.026	<0.001	0.254	<0.001
Hl (cm)	0.016	<0.05	0.056	<0.001	0.169	<0.001
Hb (cm)	0.08	<0.001	0.035	<0.001	0.245	<0.001
Hs (cm)	0.04	<0.001	0.042	<0.001	0.236	<0.001
Amg (cm)	0.001	0.991	0.041	<0.001	0.008	<0.03
Ama (cm²)	0.001	0.945	0.040	<0.001	0.009	<0.02
Aa (cm²)	0.006	0.242	0.024	<0.001	0.016	<0.002
Afa (cm²)	0.006	0.221	0.020	<0.001	0.020	<0.001
Afi	0.007	0.219	0.003	0.301	0.040	<0.001
W-hr	0.088	<0.001	0.011	<0.001	0.066	<0.001
% Bf	0.025	<0.002	0.033	<0.001	0.142	<0.001
%Lbm	0.025	<0.002	0.033	<0.001	0.142	<0.001

Table 4.12: Linear regression coefficients (Beta) of Dhgs with anthropometric variables in patients with type-2 diabetes mellitus

Variables	Diabetic males (n=251)		Diabetic females (n=325)		Combined (n=576)	
	Beta	t	Beta	t	Beta	t
Ndhgs(kg)	0.884	32.32**	0.878	31.1**	0.948	12.68**
Age (years)	-0.161	3.719**	-0.135	5.73**	-0.058	2.029**
Hv (cm)	0.098	1.545	0.174	4.122**	0.370	16.99**
Bw (kg)	0.080	0.028	0.091	4.821**	0.185	9.987**
BMI (kg/m²)	0.221	2.381*	0.163	3.322**	0.012	0.216
Uac (cm)	0.119	1.305	0.164	2.943**	0.202	3.148**
Wc (cm)	0.105	3.141	0.046	2.345**	0.127	5.679**
Hc (cm)	0.007	0.198	0.031	1.476	0.050	2.201*
Bsf (mm)	-0.033	0.655	0.076	2.611**	-0.079	2.347*
Tsf (mm)	0.009	0.208	0.109	3.871**	-0.045	1.416
Ual (cm)	0.360	1.668	0.414	3.313**	1.268	11.220**
Fal (cm)	-0.083	0.390	0.193	1.813*	0.827	7.180**
Tal (cm)	0.389	4.380**	0.208	2.958**	0.709	13.567**
Hl (cm)	0.770	1.916	0.739	4.407**	1.916	10.487**
Hb (cm)	2.643	4.370**	1.397	3.448**	4.461	13.242**
Hs (cm)	0.780	3.260**	0.594	3.777**	1.683	12.916**
Amg (cm)	-0.001	0.007	0.037	3.752**	-0.023	2.111*
Ama (cm²)	-0.001	0.021	0.046	3.70**	-0.034	2.313*
Aa (cm²)	0.002	1.172	0.003	2.84**	0.004	3.045**
Afa (cm²)	0.002	1.227	0.003	2.624**	0.004	3.393**
Afi	18.625	1.232	-9.345	1.034	46.75	4.467**
W-hr	24.126	4.546**	7.030	1.968**	23.820	6.196**
% Bf	0.165	2.381*	0.119	3.320**	-0.264	9.458**
% Lbm	-0.165	2.381**	-0.119	3.320**	0.264	9.458**

* indicates p<0.05; ** indicates p<0.001

Table 4.13: Step-down multiple regression analysis of Dhgs with anthropometric variables in diabetic males (n=251)

Variables	B	Beta	S.E	t-value	p-value
Ndhgs (kg)	0.868	0.895	0.026	32.288	**<0.001**
Age (years)	-0.032	-0.050	0.018	1.807	**<0.05**
Bsf (mm)	-0.128	0.040	-0.172	3.240	**<0.001**
Tsf (mm)	0.132	0.161	0.190	3.590	**<0.001**
Hl (cm)	0.413	0.026	0.069	2.551	**<0.01**
R^2		0.847			**<0.001**

Table 4.14: Step-down multiple regression analysis of Dhgs with anthropometric variables in diabetic females (n=325)

Variables	B	Beta	S.E	t-value	p-value
Ndhgs (kg)	0.833	0.821	0.030	27.002	**<0.001**
Age (years)	-0.024	-0.054	0.012	1.907	**<0.05**
Hv (cm)	0.248	0.318	0.146	1.695	**<0.05**
Bw (kg)	-0.260	-0.735	0.166	1.572	0.177
BMI (kg/m²)	0.700	0.777	0.404	1.731	0.084
Wc (cm)	-0.366	-1.019	0.197	1.856	0.064
Hc (cm)	0.302	0.792	0.175	1.718	0.086
Fal (cm)	-0.123	-0.641	0.063	1.953	**<0.05**
Hl (cm)	0.288	0.093	0.094	3.067	**<0.002**
Amg (cm)	0.010	0.059	0.006	1.626	0.104
W-hr	36.784	0.570	20.311	1.811	0.071
R^2		0.772			**<0.001**

Table 4.15: Step-down multiple regression analysis of Dhgs with selected anthropometric variables in patients with type-2 diabetes mellitus (n=576)

Variables	B	Beta	S.E	t-value	p-value
Dhgs (kg)	0.872	0.857	0.018	46.21	<0.001
Age	-0.019	-0.028	0.010	-1.868	0.06
Hv	0.063	0.1009	0.014	4.260	<0.001
Uac	0.051	0.0344	0.030	1.717	0.086
Bsf	-0.053	-0.068	0.024	-2.202	<0.028
Fal	-0.123	-0.044	0.054	-2.255	<0.024
Hl	0.327	0.070	0.085	3.841	<0.001
Ama	0.021	0.063	0.009	2.312	<0.02
R^2	0.883				<0.001

Table 4.16: Multiple regression of Dhgs with anthropometric variables in diabetic males

Variables	B	Beta	S.E	t-value	p-value
Ndhgs (kg)	0.854	0.88	0.032	27.056	<0.001
Age (Years)	-0.038	-0.058	0.02	1.93	<0.050
Hv (cm)	-0.004	-0.004	0.201	0.02	0.984
Bw (kg)	0.021	0.049	0.226	0.093	0.926
Uac (cm)	0.154	0.114	0.51	0.302	0.763
Wc (cm)	-0.03	-0.06	0.261	0.115	0.909
Hc (cm)	0.039	0.069	0.237	0.165	0.869
Bsf (mm)	-0.136	-0.182	0.046	2.942	<0.004
Ual (cm)	0.097	0.031	0.149	0.649	0.517
Fal (cm)	-0.082	-0.026	0.139	0.59	0.556
Tal (cm)	-0.02	-0.015	0.063	0.32	0.749
Hl (cm)	0.337	0.057	0.229	1.472	0.143
Hb (cm)	-0.067	-0.007	0.359	0.188	0.851
Hs (cm)	0.094	0.026	0.134	0.697	0.487
Ama (cm^2)	0.055	0.172	0.04	1.367	0.173
Aa (cm^2)	-0.001	-0.05	0.009	0.151	0.88
Afi	3.831	0.017	25.561	0.15	0.881
W-hr	6.479	0.08	27.575	0.235	0.814
% Lbm	0.081	0.078	0.498	0.162	0.872
R^2	0.852				<0.001

Table 4.17: Multiple regression of Dhgs with anthropometric variables in diabetic females

Variables	B	Beta	S.E	t-value	p-value
Ndhgs (kg)	0.836	0.824	0.032	26.261	**<0.001**
Age (years)	-0.023	-0.053	0.013	1.798	0.073
Hv (cms)	0.259	0.333	0.152	1.711	0.088
Bw (kg)	-0.257	-0.724	0.171	1.505	0.133
BMI (kg/m²)	0.306	0.34	0.893	0.343	0.732
Uac (cm)	0.343	0.336	0.48	0.714	0.476
Wc (cm)	-0.377	-1.049	0.204	1.848	0.066
Hc (cm)	0.313	0.821	0.181	1.725	0.086
Bsf (mm)	-0.009	-0.018	0.03	0.311	0.756
Tsf (mm)	-0.027	-0.051	0.09	0.295	0.768
Ual (cm)	-0.108	-0.047	0.105	1.028	0.305
Fal (cm)	-0.093	-0.048	0.073	1.267	0.206
Tal (cm)	0.004	0.003	0.05	0.075	0.941
Hl (cm)	0.339	0.109	0.116	2.936	**<0.004**
Hb (cm)	0.077	0.01	0.265	0.293	0.77
Hs (cm)	-0.096	-0.033	0.103	0.933	0.351
Afa (cm²)	-0.004	-0.202	0.008	0.563	0.574
Afi	-15.029	-0.092	21.377	0.703	0.483
W-hr	37.851	0.586	20.996	1.803	0.072
% Lbm	-0.272	-0.414	0.579	0.469	0.639
R^2	0.774				**<0.001**

Table 4.18: Multiple regression of Dhgs with anthropometric variables in patients with type-2 diabetes mellitus

Variables	B	Beta	S.E	t-value	p-value
Ndhgs (kg)	0.847	0.832	0.021	39.729	**<0.001**
Age (years)	-0.025	-0.038	0.011	2.365	**<0.018**
Hv (cms)	0.064	0.102	0.071	0.902	0.368
Bw (kg)	-0.038	-0.081	0.076	0.499	0.618
BMI (kg/m²)	0.278	0.201	0.205	1.357	0.175
Uac (cm)	0.279	0.185	0.321	0.874	0.384
Wc (cm)	-0.148	-0.277	0.154	0.965	0.335
Hc (cm)	0.118	0.201	0.137	0.862	0.389
Bsf (mm)	-0.053	-0.067	0.025	2.117	**<0.035**
Ual (cm)	-0.053	-0.018	0.084	-0.632	0.529
Fal (cm)	-0.084	-0.03	0.066	1.275	0.203
Tal (cm)	0.018	0.013	0.037	0.481	0.631
Hl (cm)	0.282	0.06	0.101	2.783	**<0.006**
Hb (cm)	0.094	0.01	0.21	0.447	0.655
Hs (cm)	-0.011	-0.003	0.08	0.142	0.887
Ama (cm²)	0.013	0.038	0.024	0.538	0.591
Aa (cm²)	-0.004	-0.117	0.006	0.641	0.522
Afi	-9.111	-0.039	15.382	0.592	0.554
W-hr	15.596	0.169	15.947	0.978	0.329
% Lbm	0.106	0.151	0.035	3.011	**<0.003**
R^2	0.886				**<0.001**

Table 4.19: Correlations of Ndhgs with selected anthropometric variables in patients with type-2 diabetes mellitus

Variables	Diabetic males (n=251)		Diabetic females (n=325)		Combined (n=576)	
	r	p	r	p	r	p
Age (years)	-0.217	<0.001	-0.303	<0.001	-0.086	<0.046
Hv (cm)	0.037	0.586	0.247	<0.001	0.557	<0.001
Bw (kg)	0.143	<0.035	0.235	<0.001	0.363	<0.001
BMI (kg/m²)	0.144	<0.035	0.144	<0.009	-0.004	0.933
Uac (cm)	0.048	0.481	0.143	<0.01	0.111	<0.01
Wc (cm)	0.183	<0.007	0.132	<0.017	0.227	<0.001
Hc (cm)	-0.024	0.723	0.063	0.256	0.071	0.101
Bsf (mm)	-0.054	0.432	0.106	0.056	-0.113	<0.009
Tsf (mm)	-0.044	0.520	0.167	<0.002	-0.093	<0.031
Ual (cm)	0.082	0.228	0.223	<0.001	0.426	<0.001
Fal (cm)	-0.069	0.312	0.129	<0.02	0.280	<0.001
Tal (cm)	0.265	<0.001	0.187	<0.001	0.493	<0.001
Hl (cm)	0.06	0.382	0.167	<0.003	0.353	<0.001
Hb (cm)	0.252	<0.001	0.149	<0.007	0.461	<0.001
Hs (cm)	0.173	<0.011	0.202	<0.001	0.457	<0.001
Amg (cm)	0.058	0.40	0.160	<0.004	-0.121	<0.005
Ama (cm²)	-0.061	0.37	0.157	<0.005	-0.130	<0.003
Aa (cm²)	0.041	0.549	0.136	<0.014	0.107	<0.013
Afa (cm²)	0.048	0.482	0.128	<0.021	0.123	<0.004
Afi	0.107	0.119	-0.026	0.645	0.214	<0.001
W-hr	0.302	<0.001	0.137	<0.013	0.272	<0.001
% Bf	0.144	<0.035	0.144	<0.009	-0.369	<0.001
% Lbm	-0.144	<0.035	-0.144	<0.009	0.369	<0.001

Table 4.20: Linear regression of Ndhgs with anthropometric variables in patients with type-2 diabetes mellitus

Variables	Diabetic males (n=251)		Diabetic females (n=325)		Combined (n=576)	
	R^2	p	R^2	p	R^2	p
Dhgs (kg)	0.83	<0.001	0.75	<0.001	0.869	<0.001
Age (years)	0.047	<0.001	0.091	<0.001	0.007	<0.04
Hv (cm)	0.001	0.586	0.060	<0.001	0.310	<0.001
Bw (kg)	0.020	<0.035	0.055	<0.001	0.131	<0.001
BMI (kg/m²)	0.020	<0.035	0.020	<0.001	0.001	0.933
Uac (cm)	0.002	0.481	0.020	<0.017	0.012	<0.009
Wc (cm)	0.034	<0.001	0.017	0.256	0.051	<0.001
Hc (cm)	0.005	0.723	0.003	0.056	0.004	0.101
Bsf (mm)	0.002	0.432	0.011	<0.002	0.012	<0.008
Tsf (mm)	0.001	0.519	0.027	<0.001	0.008	<0.03
Ual (cm)	0.006	0.227	0.05	<0.001	0.181	<0.001
Fal (cm)	0.004	0.312	0.016	<0.001	0.078	<0.001
Tal (cm)	0.070	<0.001	0.03	<0.001	0.242	<0.001
Hl (cm)	0.003	0.382	0.027	<0.001	0.124	<0.001
Hb (cm)	0.063	<0.001	0.022	<0.001	0.212	<0.001
Hs (cm)	0.02	<0.01	0.040	<0.001	0.209	<0.001
Amg (cm)	0.003	0.400	0.025	<0.001	0.614	<0.004
Ama (cm²)	0.003	0.400	0.024	<0.001	0.016	<0.002
Aa (cm²)	0.003	0.369	0.018	<0.001	0.011	<0.013
Afa (cm²)	0.002	0.482	0.016	<0.001	0.015	<0.004
Afi	0.011	0.118	0.006	0.644	0.045	<0.001
W-hr	0.091	<0.001	0.018	<0.001	0.073	<0.001
% Bf	0.020	<0.035	0.020	<0.001	0.136	<0.001
% Lbm	0.020	<0.035	0.020	<0.001	0.136	<0.001

Table 4.21: Linear regression coefficients (Beta) of Ndhgs with anthropometric variables in patients with type-2 diabetes mellitus

Variables	Diabetic males (n=251)		Diabetic females (n=325)		Combined (n=576)	
	Beta	t	Beta	t	Beta	t
Ndhgs(kg)	0.938	32.32**	0.853	31.13**	0.916	59.877**
Age (years)	-0.146	3.251**	-0.133	5.71**	-0.057	2.001*
Hv (cm)	0.035	0.545	0.189	4.575**	0.343	15.57**
Bw (kg)	0.063	2.116*	0.082	4.342**	0.166	9.033**
BMI (kg/m²)	0.204	2.112*	0.128	2.625**	-0.004	0.084
Uac (cm)	0.066	0.705	0.143	2.595**	0.164	2.593**
Wc (cm)	0.094	2.725**	0.047	2.398*	0.119	5.415**
Hc (cm)	-0.014	0.355	0.023	1.137	0.040	1.642
Bsf (mm)	-0.041	0.787	0.055	1.915	-0.087	2.638**
Tsf (mm)	-0.031	0.645	0.085	3.049**	-0.068	2.162*
Ual (cm)	0.269	1.210	0.504	4.117**	1.218	10.918**
Fal (cm)	-0.222	1.013	0.245	2.337*	0.771	6.784**
Tal (cm)	0.370	4.020**	0.237	3.429**	0.680	13.139**
Hl (cm)	0.365	0.876	0.510	3.041**	1.615	8.762**
Hb (cm)	2.401	3.814**	1.091	2.715**	4.076	12.047**
Hs (cm)	0.638	2.566*	0.574	3.698**	1.556	11.936
Amg (cm)	-0.014	0.843	0.028	2.907**	-0.031	2.84**
Ama (cm²)	-0.020	0.899	0.037	2.853**	-0.043	3.035**
Aa (cm²)	0.001	0.601	0.002	2.471*	0.003	2.877**
Afa (cm²)	0.001	0.704	0.002	2.317*	0.003	2.877**
Afi	24.362	1.567	-4.118	0.462	48.929	9.613**
W-hr	25.309	4.636**	8.747	2.493*	24.674	6.556**
% Bf	0.152	2.122*	0.093	2.621**	-0.254	9.215
% Lbm	-0.152	2.122*	-0.093	2.621**	0.254	9.215

* indicates p<0.05; ** indicates p<0.001

Table 4.22: Step-down multiple regression analysis of Ndhgs with anthropometric variables in diabetic males (n=251)

Variables	B	Beta	S.E	t-value	p-value
Dhgs (kg)	0.931	0.904	0.030	30.828	<0.001
Bsf (mm)	0.130	0.169	0.042	3.042	<0.002
Tsf (mm)	-0.131	-0.182	0.039	3.347	<0.001
Fal (cm)	-0.170	-0.053	0.111	1.539	0.125
Tal (cm)	0.123	0.088	0.053	2.286	<0.020
Hl (cm)	-0.461	-0.076	0.195	2.366	<0.020
R^2			0.845		<0.001

Table 4.23: Step-down multiple regression analysis of Ndhgs with anthropometric variables in diabetic females (n=325)

Variables	B	Beta	S.E	t-value	p-value
Dhgs (kg)	0.829	0.841	0.029	27.967	<0.001
Age (years)	-0.021	-0.050	0.012	1.714	0.087
Wc (cm)	0.027	0.076	0.017	1.576	0.116
Hc (cm)	-0.030	-0.080	0.018	-1.665	0.097
Ual (cm)	0.203	0.091	0.067	3.021	<0.002
Hl (cm)	-0.315	-0.103	0.105	-2.990	<0.003
Hs (cm)	0.204	0.072	0.096	2.134	<0.003
R^2			0.766		<0.001

Table 4.24: Step-down multiple regression analysis of Ndhgs with anthropometric variables in patients with type-2 diabetes mellitus (n=576)

Variables	B	Beta	S.E	t-value	p-value
Dhgs	0.901	0.917	0.018	49.137	<0.001
Wc	0.029	0.056	0.013	2.130	<0.033
Hc	-0.028	-0.50	0.015	-1.813	<0.070
Bsf	0.042	0.054	0.023	1.796	0.072
Tal	0.073	0.053	0.027	2.638	<0.008
Hl	-0.241	-0.052	0.086	-2.819	<0.005
Amg	-0.019	-0.074	0.007	-2.586	<0.009
R^2	0.875				<0.001

Table 4.25: Multiple regression of Ndhgs with anthropometric variables in diabetic males

Variables	B	Beta	S.E	t-value	p-value
Dhgs (kg)	0.923	0.896	0.034	27.05	<0.001
Age (years)	0.002	0.004	0.021	0.115	0.908
Hv (cm)	0.09	0.093	0.209	0.428	0.669
Bw (kg)	-0.101	-0.229	0.235	0.431	0.667
BMI (kg/m²)	0.383	0.27	0.693	0.553	0.581
Uac (cm)	-0.088	-0.063	0.538	0.163	0.871
Wc (cm)	-0.028	-0.053	0.272	0.101	0.919
Hc (cm)	0.004	0.007	0.246	0.017	0.986
Bsf (mm)	0.13	0.169	0.048	2.702	<0.007
Ual (cm)	-0.048	-0.015	0.155	0.308	0.758
Fal (cm)	-0.1	-0.031	0.144	0.692	0.49
Tal(cm)	0.118	0.084	0.065	1.828	0.069
Hl (cm)	-0.475	-0.078	0.237	2.003	<0.047
Hb (cm)	0.207	0.022	0.373	0.556	0.579
Hs (cm)	-0.041	-0.011	0.14	0.295	0.768
Amg (cm)	-0.055	-0.218	0.036	1.524	0.129
Afa	0.001	0.051	0.009	0.16	0.873
Afi	-10.599	-0.046	26.613	0.398	0.691
W-hr	3.519	0.042	28.671	0.123	0.902
R^2	0.848				<0.001

Table 4.26: Multiple regression of Ndhgs with anthropometric variables in diabetic females

Variables	B	Beta	S.E	t-value	p-value
Dhgs (kg)	0.83	0.842	0.032	26.261	**<0.001**
Age (years)	-0.02	-0.045	0.013	1.512	0.132
Hv (cm)	-0.157	-0.205	0.151	1.036	0.301
Bw (kg)	202	0.577	0.17	1.186	0.236
BMI (kg/m²)	253	-0.285	0.89	0.284	0.776
Uac (cm)	0.205	0.204	0.479	0.428	0.669
Wc (cm)	0.212	0.599	0.204	1.039	0.299
Hc (cm)	-0.198	-0.526	0.181	1.09	0.276
Bsf (mm)	-0.008	-0.015	0.03	0.259	0.796
Tsf (mm)	-0.004	-0.008	0.09	0.043	0.966
Ual (cm)	0.165	0.073	0.104	1.581	0.115
Fal (cm)	0.019	0.01	0.073	0.257	0.797
Tal (cm)	0.013	0.01	0.05	0.255	0.799
Hl (cm)	-0.274	-0.09	0.116	2.368	**<0.018**
Hb (cm)	-0.201	-0.027	0.263	0.763	0.446
Hs (cm)	0.197	0.069	0.103	1.919	**<0.050**
Afa (cm²)	-0.005	-0.219	0.008	0.604	0.547
Afi	4.997	0.031	21.316	0.234	0.815
W-hr	-19.172	-0.301	21.004	0.913	0.362
% Lbm	0.154	0.237	0.577	0.266	0.791
R²	0.769				**<0.001**

Table 4.27: Multiple regression of Ndhgs with anthropometric variables in patients with type-2 diabetes mellitus

Variables	B	Beta	S.E	t-value	p-value
Dhgs (kg)	0.861	0.846	0.021	41.822	**<0.001**
Age (years)	-0.139	-0.209	0.021	6.541	<0.001
Hv (cm)	0.192	0.308	0.146	1.297	0.195
Bw (kg)	-0.1??	-0.263	0.157	0.764	0.445
BMI (kg/m²)	1.2?	0.884	0.419	2.881	0.004
Uac (cm)	0.781	0.527	0.658	1.187	0.236
Wc (cm)	-0.111	-0.211	0.316	0.352	0.725
Hc (cm)	0.022	0.038	0.282	0.078	0.938
Bsf (mm)	-0.099	-0.012	0.051	0.183	0.857
Ual (cm)	0.193	0.067	0.172	1.117	0.264
Fam (cm)	-0.361	-0.131	0.134	2.682	0.008
Tal (cm)	0.262	0.192	0.076	3.452	**<0.001**
Hl (cm)	-0.195	-0.043	0.208	0.941	**0.348**
Hb (cm)	0.204	0.023	0.431	0.023	0.635
Hs (cm)	0.317	0.093	0.164	0.093	0.053
Ama (cm)	-0.023	-0.068	0.051	0.068	0.645
Aa (cm²)	-0.014	-0.463	0.012	0.463	0.227
Afi	-11.643	-0.051	31.616	0.051	0.713
W-hr	23.653	0.261	32.763	0.261	0.471
% Bf	0.473	0.682	0.069	0.682	**<0.001**
R²	0.501				**<0.001**

Table 4.28: Correlations of age with selected anthropometric variables in patients with type-2 diabetes mellitus

Variables	Diabetic males (n=251)		Diabetic females (n=325)		Combined (n=576)	
	r	p	r	p	r	p
Hv (cm)	-0.022	0.751	-0.024	0.666	0.144	**<0.001**
Bw (kg)	-0.002	0.978	-0.012	0.826	0.064	0.137
BMI (kg/m²)	0.009	0.895	0.001	0.99	-0.032	0.456
Uac (cm)	0.004	0.952	-0.002	0.973	0.012	0.78
Wc (cm)	0.063	0.353	0.055	0.319	0.090	**<0.037**
Hc (cm)	0.016	0.815	0.074	0.182	0.068	0.113
Bsf (mm)	-0.042	0.535	0.008	0.887	-0.053	0.217
Tsf (mm)	-0.029	0.669	0.003	0.952	-0.053	0.218
Ual (cm)	0.156	**<0.022**	0.013	0.818	0.159	**<0.001**
Fal (cm)	0.093	0.175	-0.007	0.903	0.105	**<0.014**
Tal (cm)	0.051	0.454	0.032	0.563	0.140	**<0.001**
Hl (cm)	-0.057	0.409	0.009	0.87	0.075	0.081
Hb (cm)	-0.119	0.082	0.007	0.893	0.066	0.128
Hs (cm)	-0.108	0.114	0.049	0.38	0.092	**<0.032**
Amg (cm)	-0.033	0.63	0.004	0.947	-0.061	0.159
Ama (cm²)	-0.035	0.613	0.004	0.939	-0.063	0.146
Aa (cm²)	0.001	0.999	-0.002	0.969	0.011	0.804
Afa(cm²)	0.003	0.964	-0.003	0.962	0.017	0.693
Afi	0.059	0.392	-0.006	0.909	0.076	0.078
W-hr	0.08	0.24	-0.011	0.85	0.057	0.187
% Bf	0.009	0.895	0.003	0.951	0.136	**<0.001**
% Lbm	-0.009	0.895	-0.003	0.951	0.136	**<0.001**

Table 4.29: Correlations of Hv with selected anthropometric variables in patients with type-2 diabetes mellitus

Variables	Diabetic males (n=251)		Diabetic females (n=325)		Combined (n=576)	
	r	p	r	p	r	p
Bw (kg)	0.408	**<0.001**	0.302	**<0.001**	0.494	**<0.001**
BMI (kg/m²)	0.003	0.967	-0.093	0.094	-0.184	**<0.001**
Uac (cm)	0.192	**<0.005**	0.091	0.103	0.127	**<0.003**
Wc (cm)	0.144	**<0.035**	0.114	**<0.04**	0.215	**<0.001**
Hc (cm)	0.292	**<0.001**	0.122	**<0.027**	0.183	**<0.001**
Bsf (mm)	0.066	0.336	0.123	**<0.026**	-0.128	**<0.003**
Tsf (mm)	0.183	**<0.007**	0.171	**<0.002**	-0.093	**<0.031**
Ual (cm)	0.552	**<0.001**	0.645	**<0.001**	0.731	**<0.001**
Fal (cm)	0.566	**<0.001**	0.526	**<0.001**	0.623	**<0.001**
Tal (cm)	0.480	**<0.001**	0.574	**<0.001**	0.711	**<0.001**
Hl (cm)	0.477	**<0.001**	0.298	**<0.001**	0.550	**<0.001**
Hb (cm)	0.317	**<0.001**	0.283	**<0.001**	0.587	**<0.001**
Hs (cm)	0.297	**<0.001**	0.304	**<0.001**	0.599	**<0.001**
Amg (cm)	0.168	**<0.014**	0.173	**<0.002**	-0.124	**<0.004**
Ama (cm²)	0.162	**<0.017**	0.173	**<0.002**	-0.133	**<0.002**
Aa (cm²)	0.188	**<0.006**	0.089	0.11	0.128	**<0.003**
Afa(cm²)	0.181	**<0.008**	0.077	0.168	0.146	**<0.001**
Afi	-0.033	0.628	-0.076	0.17	0.220	**<0.001**
W-hr	-0.148	**<0.03**	0.019	0.729	0.101	**<0.019**
% Bf	0.003	0.967	-0.093	0.095	-0.627	**<0.001**
% Lbm	0.003	0.967	0.093	0.095	0.627	**<0.001**

Table 4.30: Correlations of Bw with selected anthropometric variables in patients with type-2 diabetes mellitus

Variables	Diabetic males (n=251)		Diabetic females (n=325)		Combined (n=576)	
	r	p	r	p	r	p
BMI (kg/m²)	0.912	<0.001	0.919	<0.001	0.758	<0.001
Uac (cm)	0.728	<0.001	0.725	<0.001	0.694	<0.001
Wc (cm)	0.790	<0.001	0.724	<0.001	0.751	<0.001
Hc (cm)	0.750	<0.001	0.806	<0.001	0.753	<0.001
Bsf (mm)	0.627	<0.001	0.663	<0.001	0.500	<0.001
Tsf (mm)	0.687	<0.001	0.709	<0.001	0.544	<0.001
Ual (cm)	0.267	<0.001	0.324	<0.001	0.435	<0.001
Fal (cm)	0.236	<0.001	0.211	<0.001	0.341	<0.001
Tal (cm)	0.232	<0.001	0.213	<0.001	0.382	<0.001
Hl (cm)	0.344	<0.001	0.303	<0.001	0.425	<0.001
Hb (cm)	0.363	<0.001	0.360	<0.001	0.484	<0.001
Hs (cm)	0.319	<0.001	0.307	<0.001	0.449	<0.001
Amg (cm)	0.628	<0.001	0.656	<0.001	0.476	<0.001
Ama (cm²)	0.607	<0.001	0.636	<0.001	0.453	<0.001
Aa (cm²)	0.725	<0.001	0.732	<0.001	0.698	<0.001
Afa (cm²)	0.702	<0.001	0.706	<0.001	0.684	<0.001
Afi	-0.035	0.608	0.004	0.938	0.103	<0.017
W-hr	0.248	<0.001	0.063	0.259	0.196	<0.001
% Bf	0.912	<0.001	0.919	<0.001	0.294	<0.001
% Lbm	-0.912	<0.001	-0.919	<0.001	-0.294	<0.001

Table 4.31: Correlations of BMI with selected anthropometric variables in patients with type-2 diabetes mellitus

Variables	Diabetic males (n=251)		Diabetic females (n=325)		Combined (n=576)	
	r	p	r	p	r	p
Uac (cm)	0.712	**<0.001**	0.718	**<0.001**	0.688	**<0.001**
Wc (cm)	0.802	**<0.001**	0.709	**<0.001**	0.686	**<0.001**
Hc (cm)	0.695	**<0.001**	0.792	**<0.001**	0.723	**<0.001**
Bsf (mm)	0.658	**<0.001**	0.639	**<0.001**	0.660	**<0.001**
Tsf (mm)	0.673	**<0.001**	0.668	**<0.001**	0.682	**<0.001**
Ual (cm)	0.044	0.521	0.081	0.144	-0.046	0.289
Fal (cm)	-0.001	0.988	0.009	0.867	-0.074	0.085
Tal (cm)	0.037	0.586	-0.008	0.883	-0.097	**<0.024**
Hl (cm)	0.157	**<0.001**	0.201	**<0.001**	0.079	0.066
Hb (cm)	0.256	**<0.001**	0.265	**<0.001**	0.113	**<0.008**
Hs (cm)	0.216	**<0.001**	0.198	**<0.001**	0.062	0.147
Amg (cm)	0.615	**<0.001**	0.611	**<0.001**	0.629	**0.001**
Ama (cm^2)	0.594	**<0.001**	0.591	**<0.001**	0.610	**<0.001**
Aa (cm^2)	0.710	**<0.001**	0.726	**<0.001**	0.691	**<0.001**
Afa(cm^2)	0.687	**<0.001**	0.704	**<0.001**	-0.662	**<0.001**
Afi	-0.026	0.702	0.034	0.539	-0.047	0.274
W-hr	0.333	**<0.001**	0.057	0.306	0.132	**<0.002**
% Bf	1.000	**<0.001**	1.000	**<0.001**	0.802	**<0.001**
% Lbm	-1.000	**<0.001**	-1.000	**<0.001**	-0.802	**<0.001**

Table 4.32: Correlations of Uac with selected anthropometric variables in patients with type-2 diabetes mellitus

Variables	Diabetic males (n=251)		Diabetic females (n=325)		Combined (n=576)	
	r	p	r	p	r	p
Wc (cm)	0.664	**<0.001**	0.615	**<0.001**	0.634	**<0.001**
Hc (cm)	0.704	**<0.001**	0.700	**<0.001**	0.702	**<0.001**
Bsf (mm)	0.667	**<0.001**	0.651	**<0.001**	0.626	**<0.001**
Tsf (mm)	0.43	**<0.001**	0.657	**<0.001**	0.618	**<0.001**
Ual (cm)	0.087	0.204	0.147	**<0.008**	0.135	**<0.002**
Fal (cm)	0.130	0.055	0.058	0.294	0.103	**<0.017**
Tal (cm)	0.001	0.995	0.079	0156	0.068	0.115
Hl (cm)	0.202	**<0.003**	0.103	0.065	0.147	**<0.001**
Hb (cm)	0.175	**<0.01**	0.278	**<0.001**	0.228	**<0.001**
Hs (cm)	0.188	**<0.006**	0.138	**<0.013**	0.167	**<0.001**
Amg (cm)	0.530	**<0.001**	0.548	**<0.001**	0.505	**<0.001**
Ama (cm^2)	0.493	**<0.001**	0.512	**<0.001**	0.467	**<0.001**
Aa (cm^2)	0.995	**<0.001**	0.997	**<0.001**	0.996	**<0.001**
Afa(cm^2)	0.931	**<0.001**	0.994	**<0.001**	0.993	**<0.001**
Afi	0.332	**<0.001**	0.436	**<0.001**	0.392	**<0.001**
W-hr	0.129	0.058	0.029	0.602	0.082	0.058
% Bf	0.712	**<0.001**	0.717	**<0.001**	0.436	**<0.001**
% Lbm	-0.712	**<0.001**	-0.717	**<0.001**	-0.436	**<0.001**

Table 4.33: Correlations of Wc with selected anthropometric variables in patients with type-2 diabetes mellitus

Variables	Diabetic males (n=251)		Diabetic females (n=325)		Combined (n=576)	
	r	p	r	p	r	p
Hc (cm)	0.754	<0.001	0.819	<0.001	0.794	<0.001
Bsf (mm)	0.540	<0.001	0.522	<0.001	0.469	<0.001
Tsf (mm)	0.577	<0.001	0.564	<0.001	0.504	<0.001
Ual (cm)	0.012	0.49	0.217	<0.001	0.239	<0.001
Fal (cm)	0.047	0.061	0.072	0.196	0.130	<0.002
Tal (cm)	0.128	0.075	0.088	0.112	0.185	<0.001
Hl (cm)	0.121	<0.001	0.123	<0.026	0.186	<0.001
Hb (cm)	0.269	0.18	0.252	<0.001	0.309	<0.001
Hs (cm)	0.091	<0.001	0.122	<0.027	0.186	<0.001
Amg (cm)	0.518	<0.001	0.515	<0.001	0.443	<0.001
Ama (cm^2)	0.497	<0.001	0.497	<0.001	0.422	<0.001
Aa (cm^2)	0.657	<0.001	0.614	<0.001	0.632	<0.001
Afa(cm^2)	0.641	<0.001	0.596	<0.001	0.618	<0.001
Afi	0.056	0.41	0.077	0.169	0.118	<0.006
W-hr	0.573	<0.001	0.530	<0.001	0.561	<0.001
% Bf	0.802	<0.001	0.709	<0.001	0.365	<0.001
% Lbm	-0.802	<0.001	-0.709	<0.001	-0.365	<0.001

Table 4.34: Correlations of Hc with selected anthropometric variables in patients with type-2 diabetes mellitus

Variables	Diabetic males (n=251)		Diabetic females (n=325)		Combined (n=576)	
	r	p	r	p	r	P
Bsf (mm)	0.598	<0.001	0.628	<0.001	0.579	<0.001
Tsf (mm)	0.615	<0.001	0.643	<0.001	0.591	<0.001
Ual (cm)	0.137	<0.045	0.205	<0.001	0.198	<0.001
Fal (cm)	0.148	<0.029	0.088	0.115	0.136	<0.001
Tal (cm)	0.057	0.409	0.015	0.058	0.118	<0.006
Hl (cm)	0.162	<0.017	0.152	<0.001	0.178	<0.001
Hb (cm)	0.161	<0.018	0.245	<0.001	0.224	<0.001
Hs (cm)	0.111	0.103	0.186	<0.001	0.177	<0.001
Amg (cm)	0.553	<0.001	0.587	<0.001	0.526	<0.001
Ama (cm^2)	0.530	<0.001	0.567	<0.001	0.504	<0.001
Aa (cm^2)	0.707	<0.001	0.701	<0.001	0.703	<0.001
Afa(cm^2)	0.689	<0.001	0.680	<0.001	0.685	<0.001
Afi	0.032	0.641	0.078	0.161	0.084	<0.05
W-hr	-0.103	0.131	-0.048	0.384	-0.055	0.201
% Bf	0.695	<0.001	0.792	<0.001	0.443	<0.001
% Lbm	-0.695	<0.001	-0.792	<0.001	-0.443	<0.001

Table 4.35: Correlations of Bsf with selected anthropometric variables in patients with type-2 diabetes mellitus

Variables	Diabetic males (n=251)		Diabetic females (n=325)		Combined (n=576)	
	r	p	r	p	r	p
Tsf (mm)	0.861	**<0.001**	0.861	**<0.001**	0.868	**<0.001**
Ual (cm)	-0.005	0.939	0.137	**<0.013**	-0.053	0.214
Fal (cm)	0.012	0.856	0.091	0.102	-0.038	0.372
Tal (cm)	-0.170	**<0.012**	0.091	0.738	-0.181	**<0.001**
Hl (cm)	0.131	0.054	0.123	**<0.027**	0.008	0.845
Hb (cm)	0.057	0.405	0.188	**<0.001**	-0.012	0.785
Hs (cm)	0.027	0.694	0.099	0.076	-0.068	0.113
Amg (cm)	0.832	**<0.001**	0.837	**<0.001**	0.844	**<0.001**
Ama (cm^2)	0.820	**<0.001**	0.827	**<0.001**	0.833	**<0.001**
Aa (cm^2)	0.677	**<0.001**	0.654	**<0.001**	0.631	**<0.001**
Afa(cm^2)	0.633	**<0.001**	0.606	**<0.001**	0.579	**<0.001**
Afi	-0.293	**<0.001**	-0.217	**<0.001**	-0.298	**<0.001**
W-hr	0.072	0.293	-0.018	0.741	-0.017	0.693
% Bf	0.658	**<0.001**	0.639	**<0.001**	0.589	**<0.001**
% Lbm	-0.658	**<0.001**	-0.639	**<0.001**	-0.589	**<0.001**

Table 4.36: Correlations of Tsf with selected anthropometric variables in patients with type-2 diabetes mellitus

Variables	Diabetic males (n=251)		Diabetic females (n=325)		Combined (n=576)	
	r	p	r	p	r	p
Ual (cm)	0.046	0.502	0.198	<0.001	-0.013	0.759
Fal (cm)	0.082	0.229	0.161	<0.004	0.018	0.673
Tal (cm)	-0.061	0.37	0.100	0.071	-0.112	<0.009
Hl (cm)	0.139	<0.042	0.202	<0.001	0.051	0.236
Hb (cm)	0.11	0.109	0.285	<0.001	0.046	0.29
Hs (cm)	0.064	0.346	0.179	<0.001	-0.024	0.572
Amg (cm)	0.990	<0.001	0.991	<0.001	0.990	<0.001
Ama (cm^2)	0.983	<0.001	0.984	<0.001	0.984	<0.001
Aa (cm^2)	0.650	<0.001	0.659	<0.001	0.622	<0.001
Afa (cm^2)	0.591	<0.001	0.598	<0.001	0.555	<0.001
Afi	-0.477	<0.001	-0.365	<0.001	-0.451	<0.001
W-hr	0.107	0.116	0.032	0.56	0.025	0.563
% Bf	0.673	<0.001	0.667	<0.001	0.609	<0.001
% Lbm	-0.673	<0.001	-0.667	<0.001	0.609	<0.001

Table 4.37: Correlations of Ual with selected anthropometric variables in patients with type-2 diabetes mellitus

Variables	Diabetic males (n=251)		Diabetic females (n=325)		Combined (n=576)	
	r	p	r	p	r	p
Fal (cm)	0.720	<0.001	0.656	<0.001	0.744	<0.001
Tal (cm)	0.660	<0.001	0.653	<0.001	0.756	<0.001
Hl (cm)	0.344	<0.001	0.360	<0.001	0.506	<0.001
Hb (cm)	0.325	<0.001	0.305	<0.001	0.512	<0.001
Hs (cm)	0.314	<0.001	0.257	<0.001	0.496	<0.001
Amg (cm)	0.035	0.607	0.193	<0.001	-0.038	0.376
Ama (cm^2)	0.031	0.667	0.191	<0.001	-0.046	0.288
Aa (cm^2)	0.08	0.243	0.145	<0.009	0.132	<0.002
Afa(cm^2)	0.08	0.24	0.133	<0.0016	0.142	<0.001
Afi	0.043	0.526	-0.056	0.313	0.152	<0.001
W-hr	-0.008	0.904	0.074	0.185	0.119	0.005
% Bf	0.044	0.521	0.083	0.137	-0.357	<0.001
% Lbm	-0.044	0.521	-0.083	0.137	0.357	<0.001

Table 4.38: Correlations of Fal with selected anthropometric variables in patients with type-2 diabetes mellitus

Variables	Diabetic males (n=251)		Diabetic females (n=325)		Combined (n=576)	
	r	p	r	p	r	p
Tal (cm)	0.560	**<0.001**	0.511	**<0.001**	0.560	**<0.001**
Hl (cm)	0.375	**<0.001**	0.339	**<0.001**	0.375	**<0.001**
Hb (cm)	-0.230	**<0.001**	0.275	**<0.001**	0.230	**<0.001**
Hs (cm)	0.293	**<0.001**	0.266	**<0.001**	0.293	**<0.001**
Amg (cm)	-0.057	0.325	0.168	**<0.002**	0.067	0.325
Ama (cm^2)	0.062	0.364	0.169	**<0.002**	0.062	0.364
Aa (cm^2)	0.131	0.055	0.058	0.295	0.131	0.055
Afa(cm^2)	0.131	0.055	0.045	**<0.416**	0.131	0.055
Afi	0.038	0.58	-0.125	<0.024	0.038	0.58
W-hr	-0.118	0.085	0.001	0.98	-0.118	0.085
% Bf	-0.001	0.988	0.011	**0.842**	-0.001	0.988
% Lbm	0.001	0.988	-0.011	**0.842**	0.001	0.988

Table 4.39: Correlations of Tal with selected anthropometric variables in patients with type-2 diabetes mellitus

Variables	Diabetic males (n=251)		Diabetic females (n=325)		Combined (n=576)	
	r	p	r	p	r	p
Hl (cm)	0.464	<0.001	0.353	<0.001	0.535	<0.001
Hb (cm)	0.459	<0.001	0.337	<0.001	0.580	<0.001
Hs (cm)	0.395	<0.001	0.340	<0.001	0.565	<0.001
Amg (cm)	-0.068	0.321	0.097	0.082	-0.135	<0.002
Ama (cm^2)	-0.07	0.305	0.095	0.086	-0.142	0.126
Aa (cm^2)	-0.006	0.928	0.078	0.159	0.066	<0.001
Afa(cm^2)	0.001	0.997	0.073	0.189	0.082	0.057
Afi	0.102	0.135	-0.022	0.694	0.201	<0.001
W-hr	0.109	0.109	-0.004	0.937	0.134	<0.002
% Bf	0.037	0.586	-0.006	0.911	-0.409	<0.001
% Lbm	-0.037	0.586	0.006	0.911	0.409	<0.001

Table 4.40: Correlations of Hl with selected anthropometric variables in patients with type-2 diabetes mellitus

Variables	Diabetic males (n=251)		Diabetic females (n=325)		Combined (n=576)	
	r	p	r	p	r	p
Hb (cm)	0.501	<0.001	0.533	<0.001	0.627	<0.001
Hs (cm)	0.492	<0.001	0.564	<0.001	0.641	<0.001
Amg (cm)	0.117	0.087	0.205	<0.001	0.03	0.485
Ama (cm^2)	0.11	<0.004	0.206	<0.001	0.024	0.581
Aa (cm^2)	0.195	<0.004	0.106	0.055	0.148	<0.001
Afa(cm^2)	0.193	<0.001	0.092	0.097	0.152	<0.001
Afi	0.053	0.442	-0.125	<0.024	0.082	0.058
W-hr	-0.021	0.754	-0.009	<0.872	0.061	0.154
% Bf	0.157	<0.021	0.201	<0.001	-0.218	<0.001
% Lbm	-0.157	<0.021	-0.201	<0.001	0.218	<0.001

Table 4.41: Correlations of Hb with selected anthropometric variables in patients with type-2 diabetes mellitus

Variables	Diabetic males (n=251)		Diabetic females (n=325)		Combined (n=576)	
	r	p	r	p	r	p
Hs (cm)	0.548	**<0.001**	0.477	**<0.001**	0.657	**<0.001**
Amg (cm)	0.089	0.191	0.266	**<0.001**	0.01	0.815
Ama (cm^2)	0.082	**<0.228**	0.259	**<0.001**	0.001	0.983
Aa (cm^2)	0.163	**<0.017**	0.271	**<0.001**	0.221	**<0.001**
Afa(cm^2)	0.162	**<0.017**	0.259	**<0.001**	0.230	**<0.001**
Afi	0.108	0.114	0.015	0.783	0.209	**<0.001**
W-hr	0.194	**<0.004**	0.082	0.138	0.198	**<0.001**
% Bf	0.256	**<0.001**	0.265	**<0.001**	-0.250	**<0.001**
% Lbm	-0.256	**<0.001**	-0.265	**<0.001**	0.250	**<0.001**

Table 4.42: Correlations of Hs with selected anthropometric variables in patients with type-2 diabetes mellitus

Variables	Diabetic males (n=251)		Diabetic females (n=325)		Combined (n=576)	
	r	p	r	p	r	p
Amg (cm)	0.037	0.588	0.173	**<0.002**	-0.056	0.193
Ama (cm^2)	0.028	0.68	0.171	**<0.002**	-0.66	0.128
Aa (cm^2)	0.177	**<0.009**	0.139	**<0.012**	0.164	**<0.001**
Afa(cm^2)	0.182	**<0.007**	0.130	**<0.019**	0.177	**<0.001**
Afi	0.128	0.60	-0.058	0.301	0.188	**<0.001**
W-hr	-0.019	0.78	-0.059	0.292	0.057	0.188
% Bf	0.216	**<0.001**	0.198	**<0.001**	-0.294	**<0.001**
% Lbm	-0.216	**<0.001**	-0.198	**<0.001**	0.294	**<0.001**

Table 4.43: Correlations of Amg with selected anthropometric variables in patients with type-2 diabetes mellitus

Variables	Diabetic males (n=251)		Diabetic females (n=325)		Combined (n=576)	
	r	p	r	p	r	p
Ama (cm^2)	0.999	<0.001	0.999	<0.001	0.999	<0.001
Aa (cm^2)	0.539	<0.001	0.552	<0.001	0.509	<0.001
Afa(cm^2)	0.473	<0.001	0.484	<0.001	0.436	<0.001
Afi	-0.588	<0.001	-0.483	<0.001	-0.565	<0.001
W-hr	0.095	<0.164	0.031	0.575	0.013	0.758
% Bf	0.615	<0.001	0.611	<0.001	0.593	<0.001
% Lbm	-0.615	<0.001	-0.611	<0.001	-0.593	<0.001

Table 4.44: Correlations of Ama with selected anthropometric variables in patients with type-2 diabetes mellitus

Variables	Diabetic males (n=251)		Diabetic females (n=325)		Combined (n=576)	
	r	p	r	p	r	p
Aa (cm^2)	0.502	<0.001	0.516	<0.001	0.472	<0.001
Afa(cm^2)	0.434	<0.001	0.447	<0.001	0.392	<0.001
Afi	-0.621	<0.001	-0.518	<0.001	-0.597	<0.001
W-hr	0.091	0.182	0.03	0.589	0.0009	0.827
% Bf	0.594	<0.001	0.591	<0.001	0.586	<0.001
% Lbm	-0.594	<0.001	-0.591	<0.001	-0.586	<0.001

Table 4.45: Correlations of Aa with selected anthropometric variables in patients with type-2 diabetes mellitus

Variables	Diabetic males (n=251)		Diabetic females (n=325)		Combined (n=576)	
	r	p	r	p	r	p
Afa(cm^2)	0.997	<0.001	0.997	<0.001	0.398	<0.001
Afi	0.309	<0.001	0.420	<0.001	-0.597	<0.001
W-hr	0.114	0.094	0.025	0.651	0.009	0.827
% Bf	0.710	<0.001	0.725	<0.001	0.586	<0.001
% Lbm	-0.710	<0.001	-0.725	<0.001	-0.586	<0.001

Table 4.46: Correlations of Afa with selected anthropometric variables in patients with type-2 diabetes mellitus

Variables	Diabetic males (n=251)		Diabetic females (n=325)		Combined (n=576)	
	r	p	r	p	r	p
Afi	0.377	<0.001	0.487	<0.001	0.444	<0.001
W-hr	0.111	0.104	0.024	0.672	0.076	0.076
% Bf	0.687	<0.001	0.703	<0.001	0.399	<0.001
% Lbm	-0.687	<0.001	-0.703	<0.001	-0.399	<0.001

Table 4.47: Correlations of Afi with selected anthropometric variables in patients with type-2 diabetes mellitus

Variables	Diabetic males (n=251)		Diabetic females (n=325)		Combined (n=576)	
	r	p	r	p	r	p
W-hr	0.046	0.497	0.012	0.83	0.075	0.082
% Bf	-0.026	0.702	0.034	0.543	-0.218	**<0.001**
% Lbm	0.026	0.702	-0.034	0.543	0.218	**<0.001**

Table 4.48: Correlations of W-hr with selected anthropometric variables in patients with type-2 diabetes mellitus

Variables	Diabetic males (n=251)		Diabetic females (n=325)		Combined (n=576)	
	r	p	r	p	r	p
% Bf	0.333	**<0.001**	0.058	0.297	-0.009	0.841
% Lbm	-0.333	**<0.001**	-0.058	0.297	0.009	0.841

Table 4.49: Correlations of % Bf with % Lbm in patients with type-2 diabetes mellitus

Variables	Diabetic males (n=251)		Diabetic females (n=325)		Combined (n=576)	
	r	p	r	p	r	p
% Lbm	-1.000	**<0.001**	-1.000	**<0.001**	-1.000	**<0.001**

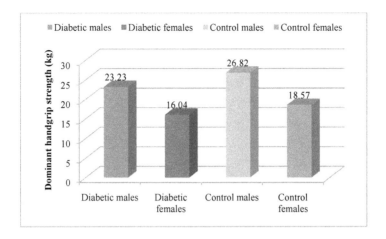

Fig. 4.1

Comparison of Dhgs (kg) and selected anthropometric variables in patients with type-2 diabetes mellitus and controls

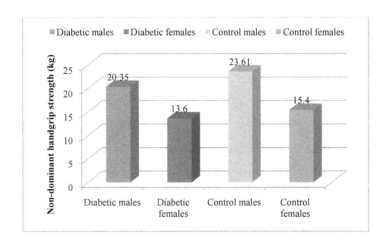

Fig. 4.2

Comparison of Ndhgs (kg) and selected anthropometric variables in patients with type-2 diabetes mellitus and controls

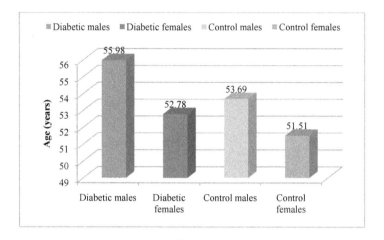

Fig. 4.3

Comparison of age (years) and selected anthropometric variables in patients with type-2 diabetes mellitus and controls

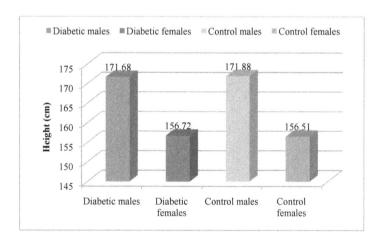

Fig. 4.4

Comparison of Hv (cm) and selected anthropometric variables in patients with type-2 diabetes mellitus and controls

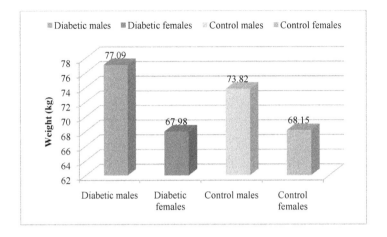

Fig. 4.5

Comparison of Bw (kg) and selected anthropometric variables in patients with type-2 diabetes mellitus and controls

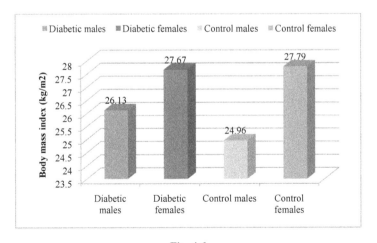

Fig. 4.6

Comparison of BMI (kg/m²) and selected anthropometric variables in patients with type-2 diabetes mellitus and controls

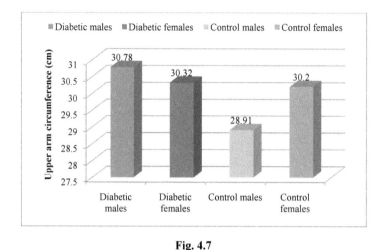

Fig. 4.7

Comparison of Uac (cm) and selected anthropometric variables in patients with type-2 diabetes mellitus and controls

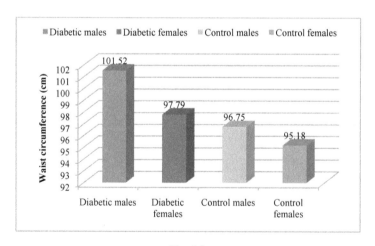

Fig. 4.8

Comparison of Wc (cm) and selected anthropometric variables in patients with type-2 diabetes mellitus and controls

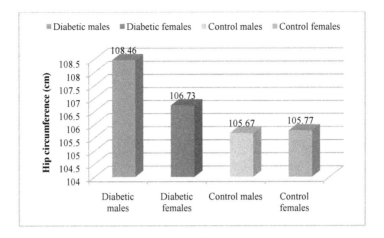

Fig. 4.9

Comparison of Hc (cm) and selected anthropometric variables in patients with type-2 diabetes mellitus and controls

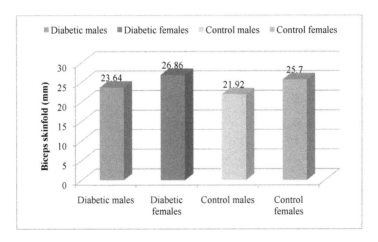

Fig. 4.10

Comparison of Bsf (mm) and selected anthropometric variables in patients with type-2 diabetes mellitus and controls

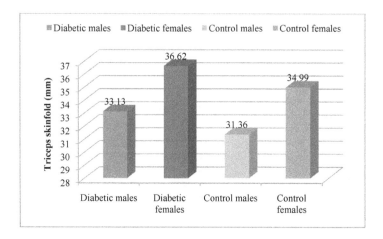

Fig. 4.11

Comparison of Tsf (mm) and selected anthropometric variables in patients with type-2 diabetes mellitus and controls

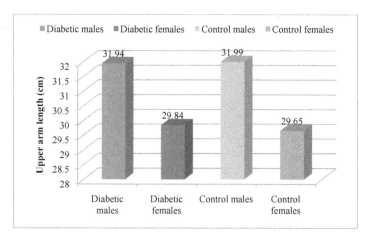

Fig. 4.12

Comparison of Ual (cm) and selected anthropometric variables in patients with type-2 diabetes mellitus and controls

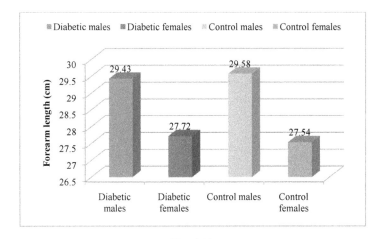

Fig. 4.13

Comparison of Fal (cm) and selected anthropometric variables in patients with type-2 diabetes mellitus and controls

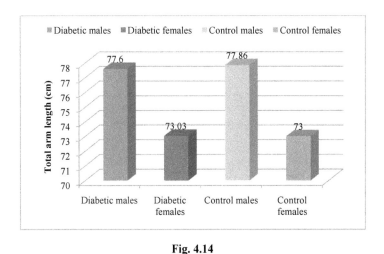

Fig. 4.14

Comparison of Tal (cm) and selected anthropometric variables in patients with type-2 diabetes mellitus and controls

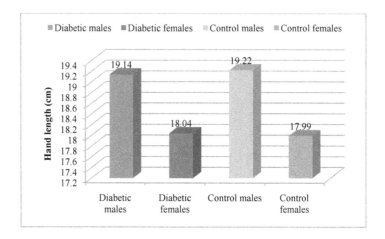

Fig. 4.15

Comparison of Hl (cm) and selected anthropometric variables in patients with type-2 diabetes mellitus and controls

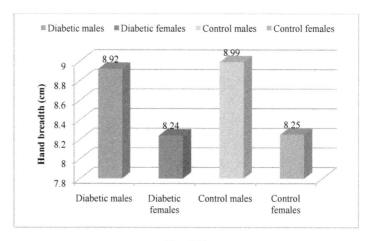

Fig. 4.16

Comparison of Hb (cm) and selected anthropometric variables in patients with type-2 diabetes mellitus and controls

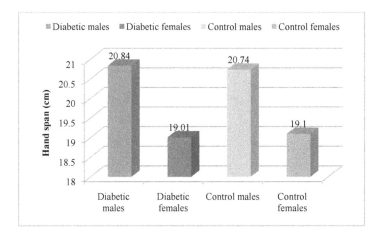

Fig. 4.17

Comparison of Hs (cm) and selected anthropometric variables in patients with type-2 diabetes mellitus and controls

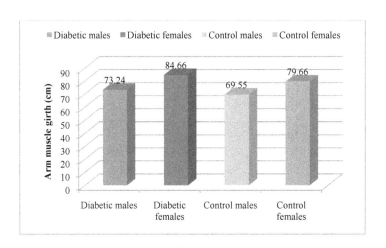

Fig. 4.18

Comparison of Amg (cm) and selected anthropometric variables in patients with type-2 diabetes mellitus and controls

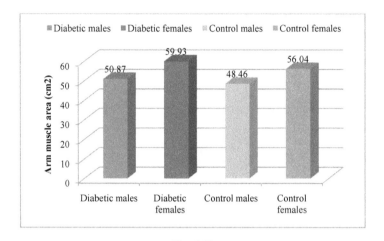

Fig. 4.19

Comparison of Ama (cm^2) and selected anthropometric variables in patients with type-2 diabetes mellitus and controls

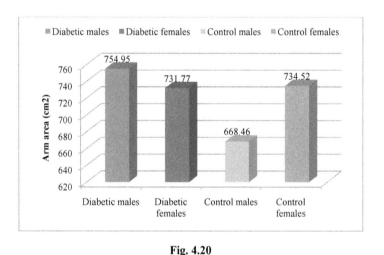

Fig. 4.20

Comparison of Aa (cm^2) and selected anthropometric variables in patients with type-2 diabetes mellitus and controls

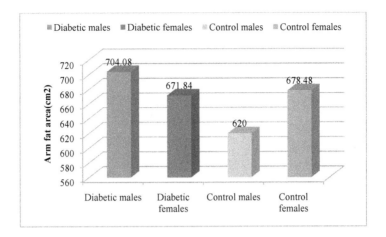

Fig. 4.21

Comparison of Afa (cm^2) and selected anthropometric variables in patients with type-2 diabetes mellitus and controls

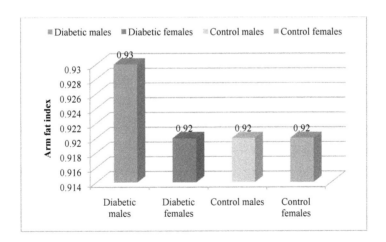

Fig. 4.22

Comparison of Afi and selected anthropometric variables in patients with type-2 diabetes mellitus and controls

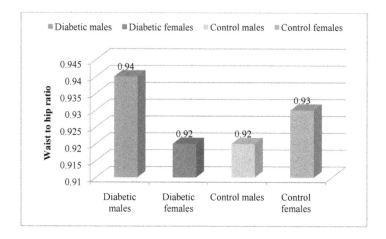

Fig. 4.23

Comparison of W-hr and selected anthropometric variables in patients with type-2 diabetes mellitus and controls

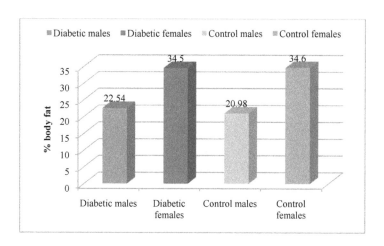

Fig. 4.24

Comparison of % Bf and selected anthropometric variables in patients with type-2 diabetes mellitus and controls

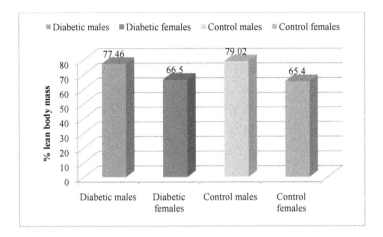

Fig. 4.25

Comparison of % Lbm and selected anthropometric variables in patients with type-2 diabetes mellitus and controls

DISCUSSION

The hand symbolizes the highly developed and distinguished musculoskeletal tool in humans, which conveys sensory information to brain about temperature, form and the texture of the object it controls (Wilk and Arrigo, 1993). Grip strength being the reliable and efficient index of functional virtue of hand, is extensively used in the assessment of hand function (Jones, 1989). Handgrip strength is the biological marker of numerous physiological systems; its assessment may be an indicator of present health status and chances of development of various chronic ailments and premature mortality (Cheung *et al.*, 2013). According to Metter *et al.* (2002) and Takata *et al.* (2007), lower handgrip strength values in middle aged and elderly subjects have been linked to premature mortality. The functional status of various systems of body including the endocrine system, can be predicted using handgrip strength values. Blackman *et al.* (2002) conducted a randomized control trial describing the increase in strength of the muscles in men, after the administration of the sex steroid and growth hormone and these findings were further reinforced by coherent study conducted by Ottenbacher *et al.* (2006). The physical attributes of an individual including all the anthropometric measurements along with bone mineral content, nutritional status and muscle strength have shown strong correlation with the handgrip strength (Copper *et al.*, 2011; Liao, 2016; Koley and Singh, 2009). Study conducted by Stenholm *et al.* (2012) described that various chronic conditions like stroke, diabetes mellitus, arthritis, coronary heart disease and chronic obstructive pulmonary disease resulted in abrupt reduction in muscular strength and subsequent reduction in handgrip strength values.

Handgrip strength values have been associated with numerous health conditions as a predictor (Angst *et al.*, 2010). In post-menopausal females, normal handgrip strength values have depicted positive association with normal bone mineral density (Karkkainen *et al.*, 2009). Monaco *et al.* (2000) recommended that handgrip strength measurement could be used as a diagnostic method for females at risk of osteoporosis. Gale *et al.* (2007) carried out a longitudinal study which reported increased mortality rates in men from cardiovascular disease and cancer, after the caliberation of muscle mass and body mass index values. Negative

113

association of handgrip strength and physical weakness has been established, even in individuals with normal values of body mass index and arm muscle circumference (Sydall *et al.*, 2003). Hand dynamometry can measure the pattern of muscle usage and determine the incidence of later life weakness and disability. Rijk *et al.* (2016) conducted a meta-analysis, which stated that in case of older adults, handgrip strength was a valid predictor of reduction in cognition, functional status and mortality. Reduction in handgrip strength values anticipated the increased dependence and decrease in intellectual abilities (Taekema *et al.*, 2010). These properties make handgrip strength as a good marker of physical fitness, social and mental health (Sallinen *et al.*, 2010).

Handgrip strength is a well accepted indicator of nutritional status, as nutritional deficiency is depicted at the earliest by decrease in functional efficiency of muscles. The study conducted by Paton *et al.* (2004) demonstrated an increase in fat-free mass and significant improvement in handgrip strength values after six weeks sip feed intervention in undernourished tuberculosis patients. Functional status is enhanced with increment in muscle function which leads to increased quality of life.

Type-2 diabetes mellitus is accompanied with poor upper limb muscle strength and muscle quality (Ezema *et al.*, 2012). Reduced muscle strength in individuals with long standing type-2 diabetes mellitus may lead to functional limitation of the limbs and physical disability. These make the day to day life of the patients with type-2 diabetes mellitus more difficult (Bardan and Laher, 2012). Reduction in sensation of the hand, due to neuropathy in long standing diabetic status, results in hindrance in activities of daily living (Cederlund *et al.*, 2009). Cardiovascular co-morbidity along with longer duration of diabetes, significantly decrease the functional health status of diabetic individuals (Grauw *et al.*, 1999). Park *et al.* (2007) showed that the loss of arm muscle mass was highest in type-2 diabetic patients with longest duration of diabetes and highest levels of HbA1c, influencing the handgrip strength values of diabetic individuals. Jekal *et al.* (2010) also stated that diabetic subjects with higher HbA1c values had considerably lower muscular endurance as compared to subjects with normal HbA1c values. Wander *et al.* (2011) suggested that lean individuals with higher muscle strength were at lower risk of developing type-2 diabetes mellitus.

Many studies have investigated the lower extremity muscle strength in patients with type-2 diabetes mellitus and identified mild weakness in distal muscles, due to diabetic neuropathy, but values of handgrip strength and pinch power in diabetic subjects are not clear in the literature, particularly in the context of Punjabi population. This study demonstrated the effect of type-2 diabetes mellitus on muscular strength by using handgrip strength as an index of muscular strength. The study also highlighted the selected anthropometric variables that have strong impact on the handgrip strength values. The determination of handgrip strength is of great significance in rehabilitation of hand. Hunt *et al.* (1985) reported that handgrip strength could predict the initial restriction of the joints of the patients with type-2 diabetes mellitus.

5.1 Comparison of Handgrip Strength and Selected Anthropometric Variables in Patients with Type-2 Diabetes Mellitus and Controls

The comparative relation between handgrip strength and selected anthropometric variables in patients with type-2 diabetes mellitus of district Amritsar of Punjab state, aged 30-65 years and age and sex matched controls was analyzed in the present study.

5.1.1 Handgrip strength of dominant and non-dominant hand

The mean handgrip strength values of dominant and non-dominant hand in the diabetic population, as reported by the present study were significantly lower ($p<0.001$) as compared to their control counterparts, which followed the findings of Leenders *et al.* (2013), Ezema *et al.* (2012) and Centinus *et al.* (2005).

In the present study, statistically significant reduction ($p≤0.001$) in dominant and non-dominant handgrip strength was reported in diabetic males in comparison to control males as earlier reported by Ibrahim (2016) and Cederlund *et al.* (2009). Significantly lower ($p<0.001$) mean values of handgrip strength of both the dominant and non-dominant hand in diabetic females were observed in comparison to control females. The above observation confirmed the results of the study conducted by Khallaf *et al.* (2014).

When comparison was made between urban and rural male diabetic patients, significant differences (p<0.01) were found in dominant handgrip strength only, but in case of female patients, no significant differences were noted. When comparison was made between urban male and female patients, and between rural male and female patients, dominant and non-dominant handgrip strength presented significant differences (p<0.001). These differences were might be due to gender differences in diabetic patients, not for habitat differences.

Helmersson *et al.* (2004) attributed the lower muscle strength in diabetic individuals then controls to increased insulin tissue resistance and hyperglycemia. In fact, such reduction in muscle strength was the result of diminished levels of sarcosomes in muscle fibres, or a decrement in the synthesis of glycogen and increment in the levels of pro-inflammatory cytokines [such as Tumour Necrosis Factor (TNF-α) and Interleukin-6]. Reduction in skeletal muscle strength can also be due to glycosylation of skeletal muscle proteins, actin and myosin. Muscle strength and performance can also be impaired due to insulin resistance as it acts as a regulator for muscle protein breakdown. Insulin is also responsible for stimulation of synthesis and maintainence of mitochondrial proteins and their functional activity (Guilet and Borie, 2005). Halvatsiotis *et al.* (2002) reported that impaired action of insulin in type-2 diabetic patients effected muscle mitochondrial protein synthesis and ATP producing key enzyme, cytochrome-c oxidase resulting in weakness and reduced endurance capacity. Reduction in the rate of glycogen synthesis in muscles, according to Peterson and Schulman (2002), may be a contributing factor for muscle weakness. Type-IIb fibres utilize muscle glycogen through anaerobic pathway and type-IIa fibres with the help of both aerobic and anaerobic metabolism (Ezema *et al.*, 2012). The oxidation of glycogen by the mitochondrion, provide energy to type-IIa fibre for sustained efforts (Centinus *et al.*, 2005). This indicates the reduction in muscle glycogen content particularly in type-IIa fibres in diabetes, effecting muscular strength. Sherman (1995) stated that poor muscle performance might also be due to poor disposal of fuel in insulin resistance state. Lesniewski *et al.* (2003) explained the relationship between subclinical neuropathic processes involving motor neurons and reduced muscle function in long standing diabetes (>6 years) with poor glycemic control. These poor glycemic control leads to reduce the quality of muscles (Ezema *et al.*, 2012).

116

About half of the type-2 diabetic patients are affected by diabetic peripheral neuropathy which is one of the most chronic complications of diabetes (Boulton *et al.*, 2005). Distal symmetrical sensorimotor polyneuropathy is a frequent neuropathic complication of diabetes that results in gradual harm to small and large fibres. The distal parts of the lower extremities are the first to be affected, resulting in stocking hypoesthesia (Boulton *et al.*, 1983), followed by distal parts of upper limbs and eventually the anterior side of the trunk. The nerve conduction velocity of median and ulnar nerves is decreased in diabetic patients in comparison to healthy individuals. Hyperglycemia is the main risk factor for diabetic neuropathy (Shaw *et al.*, 1999). Due to consistent hyperglycemia proteins undergo non-enzymatic covalent bonding with glucose, which results in alteration of their structure and functional inhibition. According to Brownlee (1992), these glycosylated proteins lead to the development of diabetic neuropathy. The increased levels of intracellular diacylglycerol due to hyperglycemia, activates protein kinase-C which causes elevated vascular permeability, reduced nitric oxide synthesis and impaired nerve regeneration (Sheetz and King, 2002). The polyol or aldose reductase pathway gets activated by increased glucose levels which results in elevated levels of sorbitol and increased activity of oxygen free radicals. The levels of dihydronicotinamide adenine dinucleotide phosphate (NADPH), nitricoxide and glutathione are decreased and osmotic stress on the cell membrane is increased. Nodal swelling and other structural changes occur due to impairment of Na^+-K^+ ATPase activity (Greene *et al.*, 1984). Azadeh *et al.* (2011) studied correlation between motor and sensory, nerve conduction velocity of the median nerve and pinch and handgrip strength in women. Park *et al.* (2006) and Lesniewski *et al.* (2003) attributed subclinical distal symmetric neuropathy for distal muscle weakness and low grip strength.

Leenders *et al.* (2013) reported rapid loss of muscle mass and muscle strength in older patients with type-2 diabetes mellitus as compared to age matched normoglycemic controls, due to blunted postprandial muscle protein synthetic response in an insulin resistant state. The loss of muscle mass and strength could also be attributed to reduction in both the number and size of myocytes (Gaster *et al.*, 2002). In type-2 diabetic individuals, low muscle attenuation values are observed which are related to decrease in oxidative enzyme activity (Simoneau *et al.*, 1995) and lower maximal aerobic capacity (Goodpaster *et al.*, 1997). Low

117

muscle attenuation in diabetic population indicates changes in muscle composition and increased fat infiltration into skeletal muscles which results in poor muscle quality (Park *et al*., 2006). Decreased muscle quality in diabetes is also associated with longer duration of diabetes and poor glycemic control due to muscle protein breakdown and inadequate energy use (Park *et al*., 2006).

The mean values of dominant and non-dominant handgrip strength presented significant differences (p<0.001) in male and female patients with type-2 diabetes mellitus. Significantly lower (p<0.001) mean values of dominant and non-dominant handgrip strength were reported in diabetic females in comparison to diabetic males, supporting the findings of Gill *et al*. (2015) and Chilima and Ismail (2001). Similar findings were also reported by Mathiowetz *et al*. (1985, 1986) who stated that males were stronger than females in both the 6-19 year old group and the adults. Crosby *et al*. (1994) and Balogun *et al*. (1991) also reported that males had higher handgrip strength than females. This difference in muscular strength in diabetic males and females could be attributed to differences in body composition between males and females as well as differences in upper body strength, as the women have the tendency of lower proportion of lean tissue distribution in the upper body as compared to men (Hurley, 1995). Males also tend to have larger muscle fibres in the upper and lower extremities as compared to women. Another reason for lower handgrip strength in diabetic females in comparison to diabetic males could be the difference related to hormonal etiologies. According to Page *et al*. (2005), the improvement in handgrip strength values of elderly men were reported after the exogenous administration of testosterone, but in contrast, no significant improvement was observed in handgrip strength values of post-menopausal women after the hormone therapy, as concluded by the study of Michael *et al*. (2010). Similar observations were made by Blackman *et al*. (2002) who confirmed the above findings through a randomized control trail, reporting significant increase in muscle strength in men after sex steroid and growth hormone intervention, but not in women. These findings suggested that sex hormones effected handgrip strength in men and women in a different manner and through different mechanisms. As compared to the contraction of type-IIa and type-IIb fibers, the contraction of type-I fibers relies more on glucose entry and metabolism, and are more responsive to insulin particularly in women lowering values of handgrip strength in diabetic

118

females. Krivickas *et al.* (2001) attributed the impaired muscle function in elderly women to age related decline in maximal unloaded shortening velocity of type-I fibers.

Significant differences in height (p≤0.001) were observed between diabetic males and diabetic females with diabetic females having lower mean value of height. This could also be possible reason of greater handgrip strength values in males. With the greater heights, arms would be proportionally longer in males, generating greater force with the greater lever arm (Chandrasekaran *et al.*, 2010). However, no significant differences in mean values of height were observed between diabetic males and control males, and diabetic females and control females.

Significant differences in body weight (p≤0.001) were observed between diabetic males and females, where diabetic males had higher mean value for body weight, following the findings of Lunde *et al.* (1972), who suggested that handgrip strength was more strongly correlated to body weight than height. Diabetic males also displayed significantly higher mean value for body weight (p≤0.001) as compared to control males. According to Schmidt and Toews (1970), grip strength increases, as body weight and height increase up to 215 lb and 75 inches respectively. No significant difference in mean values of weight was observed between diabetic females and control females.

Diabetic males reported significantly lower mean values (p≤0.001) of body mass index in comparison to control males. These might be due to the fact that long standing diabetic status caused the weight loss of the patients (Ezema *et al.*, 2012). As suggested by Hardy *et al.* (2013), higher body mass index is associated with stronger grip strength in men, explaining higher mean values of handgrip strength and body mass index in control males. But in case of diabetic females, the mean values of body mass index were comparable with mean values of control females, exhibiting no significant differences for this trait. Amongst diabetic subjects, statistically significant difference (p<0.001) was observed for body mass index, where diabetic females presented higher mean values as compared to diabetic males. In fact, Kwon (2010) suggested that females had higher body mass index in comparison to males at the time of diagnosis. Lower mean values of body mass index in females could also be explained by the inverse relationship between height and body mass index, particularly in females (Sperrin *et al.*, 2015).

5.1.2 Hand Anthropometry

The hand anthropometric characteristics included hand length, hand breadth and hand span. According to Visnapuu and Jurimae (2007), the above anthropometric evaluations are the salient hand measurements predicting handgrip strength (Visnapuu and Jurimae, 2007). Diabetic males presented lower mean values for all the above three hand anthropometric characteristics as compared to control males, though the differences were not statistically significant. In a similar fashion, diabetic females and control females exhibited comparable mean values of hand anthropometric measurements, showing no significant differences between them. Statistically significant differences (p<0.001) in the mean values of hand length, hand breadth and hand span were observed between diabetic males and diabetic females, with diabetic females having lower mean values. According to Hager-Ross and Schieber (2000), hand length is one of the most important determining factors of handgrip strength. It was reported by Mohan *et al.* (2014) that forearm circumference and hand length came out as predictors of handgrip strength after systemic regression analysis. Alahmari *et al.* (2017) accounted hand length for 25% deviation in handgrip strength values. Women are found to have smaller hands in comparison to men (Sirola *et al.*, 2008). Study conducted by Ducharme (1977) on 1400 women with United States air force, reported that due to dimensional incompatibility and improper usage in women workers, frequent complaints were presented with soldering tools, pliers and wire strippers. As hand dimensions showed sexual dimorphism with significantly higher mean values in males, they are useful parameter to discriminate sex (Varu *et al.*, 2016). The study conducted by Koley and Singh (2009) showed a strong association of handgrip strength of dominant right hand with hand length, hand breadth forearm girth.

5.1.3 Circumferential measurements

Upper arm circumference, waist circumference, hip circumference and waist to hip ratio were the circumferential measurements assessed in the study. In all these circumferential measurements, significant differences (p<0.01) were found between diabetic males and their control counterparts, showing higher mean values in diabetic males. The mean values of all the circumferential measurements in diabetic females and control females were comparable with no significant differences, except in the mean values of waist circumference where diabetic females had significantly higher (p<0.01) mean value than control females. Amongst diabetic males and females, significantly (p<0.04-0.001) lower mean values of all the circumferential measurements, except upper arm circumference were observed in diabetic females.

Circumferential measurements are considered to be the markers of central obesity and are associated with incidence of type-2 diabetes mellitus (Hartwig *et al.*, 2016). The circumferential measurements have an edge over measurements of body mass index and body weight alone, as the visceral fat tissue performs many functions, including endocrine functions (Vazquez *et al.*, 2007; Bray *et al.*, 2008). The inappropriate distribution of fat shows stronger relation with type-2 diabetes mellitus in contrast to increment in body mass index solely. According to Hartwig *et al.* (2015), waist to hip ratio is a weak indicator of incident of diabetes which might be due to its weak correlation with visceral fat in comparison to waist circumference. Hip circumference is an important element of waist to hip ratio and can act as an important indicator of visceral organs and abdominal fat (Molarius and Seidell, 1998). The study conducted by Ford *et al.* (2003) reported that males presented higher mean value of waist circumference as compared to females; the mean value of waist circumference has been reported larger than 6 cm in men than women.

5.1.4 Skinfold Measurements

The skinfold measurements included biceps and triceps skinfold to assess relation between type-2 diabetes mellitus and skinfold thickness. The values of % body fat and % lean body mass were also assessed. The biceps and triceps skinfold measurements represent subcutaneous fat distribution sequence in type-2 diabetic patients, which differs significantly from age and sex matched non-diabetic individuals (Feldman *et al.*, 1969). Diabetic males possessed significantly higher (p<0.03-0.001) mean values of biceps skinfold, triceps skinfold and % body fat, whereas, diabetic males have significantly lower mean value of % lean body mass (p<0.001) as compared to their control counterparts. The mean values of biceps skinfold, triceps skinfold, % body fat and % lean body mass did not present any significant difference in diabetic and control females. This difference could be explained by the findings that there was significant variability in skinfold compressibility among men but less corresponding variability in women skinfold compressibility due to differences in the distribution of fibrous tissue and blood vessels in the subcutaneous tissue mediated through genetic and/or hormonal differences in men and women (Mc Rae *et al.,* 2010; Himes *et al.,* 1979). Gender based differences in skinfold measurements in diabetic subjects represented significantly higher (p<0.001) mean values of biceps skinfold, triceps skinfold and % body fat, and significantly lower (p<0.001) mean value of % lean body mass in diabetic females as compared to diabetic males, following the findings of Feldman *et al.* (1969). According to them, diabetic patients were accompanied by centripetal distribution of subcutaneous fat, more in diabetic females than diabetic males.

A study conducted by Selvi *et al.* (2016) reported that skinfold thickness depended on the duration of type-2 diabetes mellitus, where increased skinfold thickness measurements at biceps and triceps were found in diabetic individuals with duration of disease of less than ten years, but reduction in skinfold thickness with duration of disease extending above ten years. It might be due to increase efflux of free fatty acids from the adipose tissue, due to absence of insulin or due to decreased sensitivity to insulin. It was also concluded in the study that skinfold thickness measurements have significant positive relation with blood pressure, and could be seen as possible indicator of possible underlying cardiovascular disease.

5.1.5   Arm Anthropometry

Arm anthropometry involved the measurements of upper arm length, forearm length, total arm length, arm muscle girth, arm muscle area, arm area, arm fat area and arm fat index. Diabetic males presented significantly higher (p<0.001) mean values of arm area, arm fat area and arm fat index as compared to control males. The mean values of rest of the measurements were also higher in diabetic males than control males, but the differences were not statistically significant. Diabetic females possessed significantly higher (p<0.01-0.001) mean values of arm muscle girth and arm muscle area in comparison to control females. Higher mean values of upper arm length, forearm length, total arm length and lower mean values of arm area and arm fat area and similar mean value of arm fat index were recorded for diabetic females as compared to control females, but once again, the differences were not statistically significant. An irregular pattern of variation for all the above parameters was observed between diabetic males and females due to physiological differences, following the findings of Kubota *et al.* (2011) and Parvatikar *et al.* (2009). Diabetic males possessed significantly higher (p<0.03-0.001) mean values of upper arm length, forearm length, total arm length, arm fat area and arm fat index as compared to diabetic females. Significantly higher (p<0.001) mean values of arm muscle girth and arm muscle area were recorded for diabetic females in comparison to diabetic males. The mean value of arm area was higher in diabetic males than diabetic females, but the differences were not statistically significant.

5.2 Correlations of Handgrip Strength with Selected Anthropometric Variables in Patients with Type-2 Diabetes Mellitus

5.2.1 Bivariate correlation

The correlations between handgrip strength and selected anthropometric variables were determined using Karl Pearson's product moment correlation coefficients. The correlations were found to be significant (p<0.035-0.001) with most of the anthropometric characteristics studied in diabetic females but with selected parameters in diabetic males. In type-2 diabetic males, significant positive correlations (p<0.018-0.001) of dominant handgrip strength were observed with non-dominant handgrip strength, body weight, body mass index, waist circumference, total arm length, hand breadth, hand span, waist to hip ratio and % body fat, and significant negative correlations (p<0.018-0.001) with age and % lean body mass. Significant positive correlations (p<0.035-0.001) of non-dominant handgrip strength in type-2 diabetic males were observed with body weight, body mass index, waist circumference, total arm length, hand breadth, hand span, waist to hip ratio and % body fat, while significant negative correlations (p<0.001) were observed with age and % lean body mass. In type-2 diabetic females, dominant handgrip strength presented significant positive correlations (p<0.019-0.001) with non-dominant handgrip strength and all the anthropometric variables, except forearm length, hip circumference and arm fat index, whereas significant negative correlations (p<0.001) were observed with age and % lean body mass. Significant positive correlations (p<0.017-0.001) of non-dominant handgrip strength in type-2 diabetic females were observed with all the anthropometric variables, except hip circumference, biceps skinfold and arm fat index, while significant negative correlations (p<0.001) were reported with age and % lean body mass.

5.2.2 Linear regression analysis

Statistically significant correlations (p<0.05-0.001) of dominant handgrip strength in diabetic males were observed with non-dominant handgrip strength, age, body weight, body mass index, waist circumference, total arm length, hand length, hand breadth, hand span, waist to hip ratio, % body fat and % lean body mass as shown by linear regression analysis. In diabetic males, non-dominant handgrip strength significantly correlated (0.035-0.001) with dominant handgrip strength, age, body weight, body mass index, waist circumference, total arm length, hand breadth, hand span, waist to hip ratio, % body fat and % lean body mass. Highly significant (p<0.02-0.001) correlations of dominant handgrip strength in diabetic females were observed with all the anthropometric characteristics studied, except hip circumference, forearm length and arm fat index. Non-dominant handgrip strength in diabetic females, showed significant correlations (p<0.02-0.001) with all the anthropometric variables studied, except hip circumference, biceps skinfold, arm fat index and waist to hip ratio.

5.2.3 Multiple regression analysis

Significant correlation (p<0.05-0.001) (R^2=0.85) of dominant handgrip strength in diabetic males was observed with selected anthropometric variables including non-dominant handgrip strength (t=27.056), age (t=0.050) and biceps skinfold (t=2.942) in multiple regression analysis. Non-dominant handgrip strength (t=26.261) and hand length (t=2.936) were the only variables that presented significant correlations (p<0.04-0.001) with dominant handgrip strength (R^2=0.774) in case of diabetic females. Multiple regression of non-dominating handgrip strength with selected anthropometric variables in diabetic males showed that only dominant handgrip strength (t=27.05), biceps skinfold (t=2.702) and hand length (t=2.003) correlated significantly (p<0.050-0.001) (R^2=0.848). In diabetic females, only dominant handgrip strength (t=26.261), hand length (t=2.368) and hand span (t=1.919) showed significant correlation (p<0.047-0.001) with non-dominant handgrip strength (R^2=0.769).

5.2.4 Step-down multiple regression analysis

Step-down multiple regression analysis showed that in diabetic males, dominant handgrip strength correlated significantly (p<0.05-0.001) (R^2=0.847) with non-dominant handgrip strength (t=32.288), age (t=1.807), biceps skinfold (t=3.240), triceps skinfold (t=3.590) and hand length (t=2.551). In diabetic females, dominant handgrip strength correlated significantly (p<0.05-0.001) (R^2=0.772) with non-dominant handgrip strength (t=27.002), age (t=1.907), height (t=1.695), forearm length (t=1.953) and hand length (t=3.067). Step-down multiple regression analysis of non-dominant handgrip strength in diabetic males showed statistically significant correlation (p<0.05-0.001) (R^2=0.845) with dominant handgrip strength (t=30.828), biceps skinfold (t=3.042), triceps skinfold (t=3.347), total arm length (t=2.286) and hand length (t=2.366). Non-dominant handgrip strength correlated significantly (p<0.003-0.001) with dominant handgrip strength (t=27.967), upper arm length (t=3.021), hand length (t=2.996) and hand span (t=2.134) (R^2=0.776) in diabetic females.

5.3 Strength of the Study

1. On the best of our knowledge, the findings of the present study are the first of its kind reporting the handgrip strength of patients with type-2 diabetes mellitus in Punjabi population.

2. The unique criteria of the study was the large sample size comprising of 576 type-2 diabetic patients and 529 controls, with no present study considering such a large number of subjects.

3. The results of the present study can be used to assess the quality of life in patients with type-2 diabetes mellitus.

4. The outcomes of this study are very important in terms of practical application involving the designing of optimal rehabilitation programme and exercise protocol for diabetic individuals.

5. The study included a large number of anthropometric variables (22 anthropometric characteristics) and studied their correlations with both

dominant and non-dominant handgrip strength, which was not done in any previous studies.

6.   The study included latest references, supporting as well as criticizing the study outcomes.

5.4   Limitations of the Study

1.   The study included the subjects only in the age group from 30-65 years.

2.   Samples were selected specifically from Amritsar, Punjab.

3.   People suffering from any other disease other than type-2 diabetes were not considered for the study.

4.   Patients having any hand injury were excluded.

SUMMARY AND CONCLUSION

INTRODUCTION

Diabetes mellitus is defined as a metabolic syndrome occurring either due to defects in insulin secretion, insulin action or both (Kumar and Clark, 2002; Beverly and Eschwege, 2003; Lindberg *et al.*, 2004). It is a heterogeneous group of disorder which results in chronic hyperglycaemia and derangements of all metabolic pathways of catabolism and anabolism of carbohydrates, lipids, proteins, minerals and water due to insulin deficiency (Shillitoe, 1988; Votey and Peters, 2004) Long standing derangements often lead to permanent or irreversible damage to body cells leading to severe diabetic complications like retinopathy (Bearse *et al.*, 2004; Hove *et al.*, 2004), neuropathy (Seki *et al.*, 2004; Moran *et al.*, 2004), nephropathy (Huang and Caramori, 2002; Shukla *et al.*, 2003) and cardiovascular complications (Svensson *et al.*, 2004; Saely *et al.*, 2004).

According to International Diabetes Federation (2013), type-2 diabetes mellitus affects 382 million people worldwide and expected to rise to 592 million by 2035. Diabetes Atlas estimates the number of persons with diabetes in India to rise from 40 million in 2007 to 70 million in 2025 earning the dubious distinction of "diabetes capital of the world". The highest number of diabetic patients by 2025 will be in India, China, and United States (King *et al.*, 1998; Ramachandran *et al.*, 2007). World Health Organization (1994) stated that rapid cultural and social dynamics, ageing populations, increasing urbanization, dietary changes, reduced physical activity and other unhealthy lifestyle and behavioural patterns have increased the incidence of diabetes mellitus particularly in developing countries.

Grip strength is a reliable and valid evaluation of hand strength and can provide an objective index of hand and upper body strength (Methot *et al.*, 2010). Handgrip strength is an established marker for conditioning and has specifically shown to be associated with overall fitness in persons with type-1 and type-2 diabetes mellitus (Wallymahmed *et al.*, 2007). Redmond *et al.* (2009) reported the strong association of weakness of hand muscles and peripheral sensory neuropathy with diabetes mellitus.

Lower handgrip strength has been linked with functional disability and premature mortality in middle-aged and elderly subjects (Metter *et al.*, 2002).

Type-2 diabetes mellitus patients are susceptible to higher disabilities in self-care tasks and daily routine activities as compared to non-diabetic subjects due to enormous hand complications (Badran *et al.*, 2012). However, lesser attention has been paid to functioning of hand in type-2 diabetes patients as compared to diabetic foot and other diabetic complications (Redmond *et al.*, 2009). To fill the void of literature related to the strength of the hand in patients with type-2 diabetes mellitus, especially in north Indian context, the present study was planned.

Aims and Objectives

The present study was conducted with the following aims:

- To evaluate handgrip strength of patients with type-2 diabetes mellitus.

- To evaluate the handgrip strength of age, sex matched controls.

- To compare the handgrip strength between the patients with type-2 diabetes mellitus and controls.

- To evaluate the sex differences for handgrip strength in patients with type-2 diabetes mellitus and controls.

- To establish correlations with handgrip strength and selected anthropometric measurements in patients with type-2 diabetes mellitus.

Hypothesis

There would be significant differences of handgrip strength between the patients with type-2 diabetes mellitus and controls age group-wise. There would be significant correlations between handgrip strength and selected anthropometric variables in patients with type-2 diabetes mellitus.

MATERIALS AND METHODS

Sample Selection

Study group consisted of 576 confirmed cases of type-2 diabetes mellitus (251 males, 325 females) with a mean duration of diabetes of more than 5 years, and 529 controls (241 males, 288 females) without any history of glucose intolerance. The subjects ranged from age group of 30-65 years. The age of the subjects was estimated from their date of birth. The subjects with any history of pain and musculoskeletal problems in the shoulder, arm or hand, documented history of trauma or brachial plexus injury, or cervical radiculopathy in the previous 6 months of the commencement of the study were excluded from the study. The consent was obtained from the subjects in written format. The study was approved by institutional ethical committee.

Methods

Procedure of estimating handgrip strength

Dominant and non-dominant handgrip strength was measured by graded digital dynamometer, manufactured by Takei Scientific Instruments Co., Ltd., Japan. The measurement of handgrip strength was done in an upright position with full extension position of elbow. The participants were asked to apply utmost pressure on the handle of the dynamometer. The procedure was repeated three times and the mean value was recorded in kg. Hand-held handgrip strength dynamometer was calibrated before each measurement.

Anthropometric measurements

As many as 22 anthropometric measurements namely height vertex, body weight, body mass index, upper arm, waist and hip circumference, biceps and triceps skinfold, upper arm, forearm and total arm length, hand length, breadth and span, arm muscle girth, arm muscle area, arm area, arm fat area, arm fat index, waist to hip ratio, % body fat and % lean body mass were taken. All the anthropometric measurements were taken on each subject, following the guidelines given by Lohmann *et al.* (1988).

RESULTS AND DISCUSSION

Comparison of handgrip strength and selected anthropometric variables in patients with type-2 diabetes mellitus

The comparative relation between handgrip strength and selected anthropometric variables in patients with type-2 diabetes mellitus of district Amritsar of Punjab state, aged 30-65 years and age and sex matched controls was analyzed in the present study. The findings revealed that mean values of handgrip strength of dominant and non-dominant hand in diabetic population were significantly lower ($p < 0.001$) as compared to normal subjects, which followed the findings of Akpinar *et al.* (2017), Leenders *et al.* (2013), Ezema *et al.* (2012) and Centinus *et al.* (2005).

In the present study, it was reported that diabetic males had significantly lower ($p < 0.001$) mean values of dominant and non-dominant handgrip strength in comparison to control males. The findings of the present study were supported by the earlier reports of Ibrahim (2016) and Cederlund *et al.* (2009). Significantly lower ($p < 0.001$) mean values of dominant and non-dominant handgrip strength were reported in diabetic females in comparison to control group, supporting the findings of Khallaf *et al.* (2014). The reduced muscle strength in patients with type-2 diabetes mellitus than controls could be due to either increased insulin tissue resistance and hyperglycaemia or decrement of glycogen synthesis which had a damaging effect on the skeletal muscles (Helmersson *et al.*, 2004).

Sex differences in handgrip strength in patients with type-2 diabetes mellitus were also observed in the present study. Significantly lower ($p < 0.001$) mean values of dominant and non-dominant handgrip strength were reported in diabetic females in comparison to diabetic males, supporting the findings of Gill *et al.* (2015) Chilima and Ismail (2001) and Mathiowetz *et al.* (1985) which attributed this difference to physiological disparities between males and females with males having greater muscle mass and strength.

When comparison was made between urban and rural male diabetic patients, significant differences ($p < 0.01$) were found in dominant handgrip strength only, but in case of female patients, no significant differences were noted. When comparison was made between urban male and female patients, and between rural male and female patients, dominant and non-dominant handgrip strength presented significant differences (p<0.001). These differences were might be due to gender differences in diabetic patients, not for habitat differences.

Significant differences (p<0.001) in height and body weight were observed between diabetic males and females where diabetic females had significantly lower mean values of both height and body weight. Diabetic males displayed significantly higher mean values of body weight (p<0.001) as compared to control males as diabetic subjects generally tend to be obese as explained by Kaye *et al.* (1991) and Harris *et al.* (1987).

Diabetic males reported significantly lower mean values (p<0.001) of body mass index in comparison to control males. Long standing diabetic status would be the reason for weight loss in the patients (Ezema *et al.*, 2012). But in case of diabetic females, the mean values of body mass index were comparable exhibiting no significant differences as compared to control females. Amongst diabetic subjects, statistically significant difference (p<0.001) was observed for body mass index, where diabetic females presented higher mean values as compared to diabetic males. In fact, Kwon (2010) suggested that females had higher body mass index values in comparison to males at the time of diagnosis of diabetes. Long standing diabetic status also affected the weight loss only in male patients.

Hand Anthropometry

Hand anthropometry consisted of measurements of hand length, hand breadth and hand span of the dominant and non-dominant hand. The mean values of all the three anthropometric measurements of hand were almost similar in diabetic males and control males with no significant difference. Similarly, between diabetic females and control females, no significant differences in mean values of hand length, hand breadth and hand span were observed. Statistically significant differences (p<0.001) prevailed between the mean values of all the three anthropometric measurements of the hand of diabetic males and females, with diabetic females having lower mean values of all the three measurements. As hand dimensions showed sexual dimorphism with significantly higher values in males, they are useful parameters to discriminate sex (Varu *et al.,* 2016).

Circumferential Measurements

Upper arm circumference, waist circumference, hip circumference and waist to hip ratio were the circumferential measurements assessed in the study. Significantly higher mean values (p<0.001) were observed in all the above mentioned circumferential measurements in diabetic males than their control counterparts. The mean values of all the circumferential measurements in diabetic females and control females were comparable with no significant difference, except for the mean values of waist circumference presenting a significantly higher (p<0.01) value in diabetic females. Amongst diabetic males and females, significantly (p<0.04-0.001) lower mean values of all the circumferential measurements were observed in diabetic females.

Skinfold Measurements

The skinfold measurements included biceps and triceps skinfold. The values of % body fat and % lean body mass were also assessed. Diabetic males possessed significantly higher (p<0.03-0.001) mean values of biceps skinfold, triceps skinfold and % body fat, whereas, significantly lower mean values of % lean body mass (p<0.001) as compared to their control counterparts. The mean values of biceps skinfold, triceps skinfold, % body fat and % lean body mass did not present any significant difference in diabetic and control females. This difference could be explained by the findings that there was significant variability in skinfold compressibility among men but less corresponding variability in women skinfold compressibility due to differences in the distribution of fibrous tissue and blood vessels in the subcutaneous tissue mediated through genetic and/or hormonal differences in men and women (Mc Rae *et al.,* 2010; Himes *et al.,* 1979). Gender based differences in skinfold measurements in diabetic subjects represented significantly higher (p<0.001) mean values of biceps skinfold, triceps skinfold and % body fat, and significantly lower (p<0.001) mean value of % lean body mass in diabetic females as compared to diabetic males.

Arm Anthropometry

Arm anthropometry involved the measurements of upper arm, forearm and total arm length, arm muscle girth, arm muscle area, arm area, arm fat area and arm fat index. Diabetic males presented significantly higher (p<0.001) mean values of arm area, arm fat area and arm fat index as compared to control males. The mean values of rest of the measurements were also higher in diabetic males than control males but significant differences were not observed. Diabetic females possessed significantly higher (p<0.01-0.001) mean values of arm muscle girth and arm muscle area in comparison to control females. Higher mean values of upper arm length, forearm length, total arm length and lower mean values of arm area and arm fat area and similar mean value of arm fat index were recorded for diabetic females as compared to control females, but significant differences were not observed. An irregular pattern of variation for all the above parameters was observed between diabetic males and females due to physiological differences, following the findings of Kubota *et al.* (2011) and Parvatikar *et al.* (2009). Diabetic males possessed significantly higher (p<0.03-0.001) mean values of upper arm length, forearm length, total arm length, arm fat area and arm fat index as compared to diabetic females. Significantly higher (p<0.001) mean values of arm muscle girth and arm muscle area were recorded for diabetic females in comparison to diabetic males. The mean value of arm area was higher in diabetic males than diabetic females but significant difference was not observed.

Correlations of handgrip strength with selected anthropometric variables in patients with type-2 diabetes mellitus

Bivariate correlation

With the Karl Pearson's product moment analyses, significant correlations (p<0.035-0.001) were found with most of the anthropometric characteristics studied in diabetic females but with selected parameters in diabetic males. Significant positive correlations (p<0.018-0.001) of dominant handgrip strength in type-2 diabetic males were observed with non-dominant handgrip strength, body weight, body mass index, waist circumference, total arm length, hand breadth, hand span, waist to hip ratio and %

body fat, and significant negative correlations (p<0.018-0.001) with age and % lean body mass. Significant positive correlations (p<0.035-0.001) of non-dominant handgrip strength in type-2 diabetic males were observed with body weight, body mass index, waist circumference, total arm length, hand breadth, hand span, waist to hip ratio and % body fat, while significant negative correlations (p<0.001) were observed with age and % lean body mass. In type-2 diabetic females, significant positive correlations (p<0.019-0.001) of dominant handgrip strength were observed with non-dominant handgrip strength and all the anthropometric variables studied, except hip circumference, forearm length and arm fat index, and significant negative correlations (p<0.001) with age and % lean body mass. Non-dominant handgrip strength in type-2 diabetic females presented significant positive correlations (p<0.017-0.001) with all the anthropometric variables studied except hip circumference, biceps skinfold and arm fat index, but age and % lean body mass presented significant negative correlations (p<0.001) with non-dominant handgrip strength in diabetic females.

Linear regression

Statistically significant correlations (p<0.05-0.001) of dominant handgrip strength in diabetic males were observed with non-dominant handgrip strength, age, body weight, body mass index, waist circumference, total arm length, hand length, hand breadth, hand span, waist to hip ratio, % body fat and % lean body mass, as shown by linear regression analysis. In diabetic males, non-dominant handgrip strength significantly correlated (p<0.035-0.001) with dominant handgrip strength, age, body weight, body mass index, waist circumference, total arm length, hand breadth and span, waist to hip ratio, % body fat and % lean body mass. Highly significant (p<0.02-0.001) correlations of dominant handgrip strength in diabetic females were observed with all the anthropometric characteristics studied, except hip circumference, forearm length and arm fat index. Non-dominating handgrip strength in diabetic females showed significant correlation (p<0.02-0.001) with all the anthropometric characteristics studied, except hip circumference, biceps skinfold, arm fat index and waist to hip ratio.

134

Multiple regression

Significant correlation (p<0.05-0.001) (R^2=0.85) of dominant handgrip strength in diabetic males was observed with selected anthropometric variables including non-dominant handgrip strength (t=27.056), age (t=0.050) and biceps skinfold (t=2.942) in multiple regression analysis. Non-dominant handgrip strength (t=26.261) and hand length (t=2.936) were the only variables that presented significant correlations (p<0.04-0.001) with dominant handgrip strength (R^2=0.774) in case of diabetic females. Multiple regression of non-dominating handgrip strength with selected anthropometric variables in diabetic males showed that only dominant handgrip strength (t=27.05), biceps skinfold (t=2.702) and hand length (t=2.003) correlated significantly (p<0.050-0.001) (R^2=0.848). In diabetic females, only dominating handgrip strength (t=26.261), hand length (t=2.368) and hand span (t=1.919) showed significant correlation (p<0.047-0.001) with non-dominating handgrip strength (R^2=0.769).

Step-down multiple regression analysis

Step-down multiple regression analysis showed that in diabetic males, dominant handgrip strength correlated significantly (p<0.05-0.001) (R^2=0.847) with non-dominant handgrip strength (t=32.288), age (t=1.807), biceps skinfold (t=3.240), triceps skinfold (t=3.590) and hand length (t=2.551). In diabetic females, dominant handgrip strength correlated significantly (p<0.05-0.001) (R^2=0.772) with non-dominant handgrip strength (t=27.002), age (t= 1.907), height (t=1.695), forearm length (t=1.953) and hand length (t=3.067). Step-down multiple regression analysis of non-dominant handgrip strength in diabetic males showed statistically significant correlation (p<0.05-0.001) (R^2=0.845) with dominant handgrip strength (t=30.828), biceps skinfold (t=3.042), triceps skinfold (t=3.347), total arm length (t=2.286) and hand length (t=2.366). Non-dominant handgrip strength correlated significantly (p<0.003-0.001) with dominant handgrip strength (t=27.967), upper arm length (t=3.021), hand length (t=2.996) and hand span (t=2.134) (R^2=0.776) in diabetic females.

135

CONCLUSIONS

1. Statistically significant differences (p<0.001) were observed in mean value of dominant and non-dominant handgrip strength in patients with type-2 diabetes mellitus and controls.

2. Diabetic males presented significantly (p<0.001) lower mean values of dominant handgrip strength as compared to control males.

3. Significantly (p<0.001) lower mean values of non-dominant handgrip strength were observed in diabetic males as compared to control males.

4. Significantly (p<0.001) lower mean values of dominant handgrip strength were reported in diabetic females in comparison to control females.

5. Diabetic females presented significantly (p<0.001) lower mean values of non-dominant handgrip strength as compared to control females.

6. Amongst diabetic males and females, significantly lower (p<0.001) mean values of dominant and non-dominant handgrip strength were observed in diabetic females.

7. In diabetic males, dominant handgrip strength presented significant positive correlations (p<0.018-0.001) with non-dominant handgrip strength, body weight, body mass index, waist circumference, total arm length, hand breadth, hand span, waist to hip ratio and % body fat.

8. Significant negative correlations of dominant handgrip strength (p<0.018-0.001) with age and % lean body mass were observed in diabetic males.

9. Non-dominant handgrip strength in diabetic males presented significant positive correlations (p<0.035-0.001) with body weight, body mass index, waist circumference, total arm length, hand breadth, hand span, waist to hip ratio and % body fat.

10. Non-dominant handgrip strength presented significant negative correlations (p<0.001) with age and % lean body mass in diabetic males.

136

11. Dominant handgrip strength in diabetic females presented significant positive correlations ($p<0.019-0.001$) with non-dominant handgrip strength, height, body weight, body mass index, upper arm circumference, biceps and triceps skinfold, upper arm and total arm length, hand length, breadth and span, arm muscle girth, arm muscle area, arm area, arm fat area, waist to hip ratio and % body fat.

12. Significant negative correlations ($p<0.001$) of dominant handgrip strength were reported with age and % lean body mass in diabetic females.

13. Non-dominant handgrip strength in type-2 diabetic females observed significant positive correlations ($p<0.017-0.001$) with height, body weight, body mass index, upper arm and waist circumference, biceps and triceps skinfold, upper arm, forearm and total arm length, hand length, breadth and span, arm muscle girth, arm muscle area, arm area, arm fat area, waist to hip ratio and % body fat.

14. Non-dominant handgrip strength reported significant negative correlations ($p<0.001$) with age and % lean body mass in diabetic females.

CPSIA information can be obtained
at www.ICGtesting.com
Printed in the USA
BVHW050932060323
659640BV00034BA/608